MARCH FORTH

MARCH FORTH

My Journey through Diagnosis, Treatment, and Recovery from Breast Cancer

MARCI A. SCHMITT

Outskirts Press, Inc.
Denver, Colorado

"Chemotherapy takes you to hell's door. It's a very rough ride on a path that slides and spirals downward, beating you down physically and mentally after each treatment. The ride allows you to escape the punishment and heal briefly in time to return for another treatment. It strips you mentally and physically to the very core of your soul and what feels like the very last second of your life. Once you have entered that second, it becomes very expansive. NOTHING else matters! You really don't know where you are going or care where you have been. You could care less if you were buck naked before the world. You just want to make it through that second so you can face the next.

It was at this point I walked and talked with God. I felt his presence helping me . . . God was my 'bridge over troubled water' when pain was all around me. . . ."

-Marci A. Schmitt

To Steve and Lindsay,

I love you,

Marci

To Corey and Clay,

I'm proud of you.
I love you.

Mom

I will survive.

__March Forth!__

CONTENTS

DISCLAIMER

Please note that this book is written about _my_ diagnosis, treatment, and recovery from breast cancer and how this journey affected _my_ life and _my_ family. The intent of this book is to inform and educate others about *my* experiences and *my* experiences solely. Maybe the insights I present in this book will help others affected by or diagnosed with breast cancer; however, any person affected by or diagnosed with breast cancer should seek the advice of a medical professional. You and only you are responsible for your actions if you choose to follow or not follow a course of treatment based on what you read in this book. I am not a medical professional. It is also not my intent to prescribe any medical treatment or advice. It is not my intent to defame medical professionals or make them look incompetent, but quite the opposite. I would like to support all the skilled medical professionals, drug manufacturers, and researchers who helped me to survive and conquer this scary diagnosis of breast cancer.

God Bless,
Marci A.Schmitt

ACKNOWLEDGMENTS

I would like to recognize, acknowledge, and commend the individuals who helped me survive my diagnosis, treatment, and recovery from breast cancer. Many friends, family members, acquaintances, and even strangers helped me *March Forth.* I could never list everyone in this short space and even if I tried, I would probably forget someone. You know who you are and my family and I thank each and every one of you. You were and are my angels!

I especially want to thank my oncologist and nurses. Every week I walked into the doctor's office and infusion room and depended upon your care. Thank you for your professionalism, encouragement, and support. You truly are unsung heroes.

I want to thank the people behind two wonderful websites that were very resourceful and informative during my journey: Pam Stephan's www.breastcancer.about.com and www.breastcancer.org. These websites provide educational and practical information for anyone affected by breast cancer.

I want to thank the people who put me in their prayer

chains and prayed for my healing and support. You all were powerful. I prayed with you and for you each night as well. I also prayed for comfort and healing for others as well as myself who were and are facing any life-threatening disease or situation.

I want to thank the meal crew for keeping my family fed. Believe me, that task was so appreciated. I also want to thank the car pool crew, who transported my sons to and from their events. In addition, I want to thank my sons' schoolteachers, who gave the extra effort to keep my sons focused on their studies.

I want to thank those individuals who were directly involved in helping me publish this book—especially my editor JoAnn Learman. Thank you for editing my book.

I want to thank Mom and Dad for instilling the fighting spirit within me. I love you both and I know you can hear me Mom.

I want to thank my sons Corey and Clay for being strong and helping the family when we were hit by this crisis. You both had to grow and mature faster than most of your peers. The reality of life hit both of you in the face and you both passed with flying colors. I love you and I am proud of you.

I want to thank Lindsay for being there for me in spirit. She also had her own mountain to climb during this ordeal. I love you and I am proud of you, too.

I want to thank my husband Steve, who was my main caregiver. You were there for the whole journey. Honey, no one can deny your effort and desire to keep me focused on surviving this scary journey. I love you.

Finally, I want to thank God. Just as you promised, you were there for me every time. Thank you for helping me to *__March Forth!__*

Marci A. Schmitt

Please visit my website at www.4marchforth.com.

INTRODUCTION

When I began writing this book, my intention was to help others who were affected by breast cancer. I had hoped to reach out and convey an understanding of what one experiences through diagnosis, treatment, and recovery. I thought if I could help at least one person with my thoughts and experiences, this book would be a success for me. Little did I know when I began writing, I would be the first person it helped.

Writing this book was positive and massive therapy for me. It allowed me to face and vent a number of feelings that I felt during my cancer diagnosis, treatment, and recovery. My good friend Ruth once told me that when we reach out to help others, God allows us to become the first benefactor. She was correct. I became the first benefactor from this book. Throughout its writing, it was my rehabilitation. Writing allowed me to begin my journey towards healing mentally and recovering physically.

To all families and survivors affected by cancer, *__March Forth!__*

Marci A. Schmitt

1
FLASHBACK

It was Friday, December 31, 2004—New Year's Eve. I began my day before dawn. It was cold and rainy. The foot of snow we'd received the previous week had melted into a muddy flood. My children were sick. It also was the beginning of the fourth day that my family was keeping a vigil over my mother.

Things were progressing very quickly for Mom. Her illness was about to win the battle. Mom was dying from breast cancer. Although breast cancer would win this battle, my mom was about to win the war. She was close to leaving us and going home to God.

Four days earlier, Mom sat in her chair at the retirement home. She and Dad had downsized, moving from a dairy farm to the retirement home just last month. Her hand cradled her face as her elbow rested on the arm of the chair. She sat in disbelief. Hospice workers had arrived. "I just can't believe I am this sick," she said. She tried valiantly to do as much as she could but was now faced with the reality that she was losing her battle to breast cancer.

Things were hectic for my family that week. We'd

had one of the biggest snowstorms that I could remember since the Blizzard of 1978. With over a foot of snow in our driveway, my vehicle was stranded in the garage. My husband Steve and I had to dig a path from our garage to the main road—approximately 50 yards. The driveway slanted uphill near the main road, creating an obstacle for our vehicles whenever we had the smallest amounts of ice or snow. I knew I had to get my car out because Mom was getting worse. I wanted to be there for her.

I also was exhausted. Dealing with Mom, my sick kids, work, my parents' move, and the holidays had spent all of my energy. *How much more hectic can things get?* I thought. I felt guilty that I could not help my mom more and that I had neglected my children enough that they were very sick.

Yesterday, Mom had suddenly started an erratic breathing pattern. I'd held her hand and repeatedly whispered into her ear, "Mom, go towards the light! Mom, go towards the light! God is waiting for you!" After two hours, she began to lie peacefully, breathing rhythmically but abnormally. I believe Mom's spirit left her during this incident.

I had gone home late Thursday night knowing my mom's spirit had passed. I wanted to tuck my young children into bed. After all, they were about to lose their grandmother and both sons were very sick.

Finally, it was Friday morning, December 31, 2004. Again, my mom lay peacefully, breathing rhythmically but abnormally. The hospice nurse came to check Mom. She stated Mom was very close to passing. I talked with the nurse briefly about the incident that had happened yesterday. I truly believed Mom's spirit left her during those few hours. The nurse agreed with me. She stated that she usually keeps those thoughts to herself but since I mentioned it, she felt others had passed that way as well. She explained that Mom had a tough, strong heart. It was like a machine that was still running but had no driver. She said we had to wait for the machine to stop.

When the doctor's office opened, I called my six-year-old son's pediatrician. Clay was very sick. He needed to see the doctor before the weekend came. His cough and cold had worsened. The doctor wanted to see him immediately. I needed to take him to the doctor but I didn't want to leave my mom. I called my husband Steve and told him I would take Clay to the doctor so he could stay with our nine-year-old son Corey who had a fever and chicken pox again.

I knew Mom would want me to take care of Clay and Corey. She loved them both, as she did all her grandchildren. She would understand if I left her. She and Clay had a special bond. Something told me to take him to the doctor. Therefore, I left to get Clay.

Clay had pneumonia, the doctor said. Treatment and medicines were given and he was to be looked over with a watchful eye. As Clay and I were walking out of the doctor's office, the call came from my sister. "Mom is starting to pass," she said.

I did not make it back to Mom's home in time to "officially" be there when she died. However, I believe I was with her when her spirit left this world to be with our Heavenly Father. She passed peacefully on Friday morning December 31, 2004. *__March Forth,__* Mom, *__March Forth!__*

2
FLASH FORWARD

It was the summer of 2008. The start of the new school year was quickly approaching. My family was returning from a vacation on the East Coast, where we had visited several historical sites and family members. As we were driving through the mountains, my thoughts returned to the previous week. I'd had a suspicious-looking mole removed from my leg. The doctor's office had called to let me know that some of the cells surrounding the mole were abnormal. However, they felt they had clipped a clear margin of good cells surrounding the mole. "No melanoma was found," the nurse said. This was comforting, but it still gave me an uneasy feeling. After all, cancer ran in my family. My mother had died from it three and a half years earlier. My father-in-law had died from it two years back. *I'm tired of that cancer! I hate it!* I briefly allowed myself to consider the possibility of having it. *I hope I __NEVER__ get it!* I thought.

I knew I had a high risk of getting cancer because of my family history, dense breasts, and my high score on the <u>Breast Cancer Risk Assessment Tool</u>. Thus, as we were driving home, my thoughts returned to the area under my left breast. It had been bothering me for some time now. I knew I had to do something about it, but again, I dismissed it and settled into being home after vacation. August quickly came and passed due to my sons' school activities and sports. My oldest son Corey was attending a new middle school and playing football for the first time. Clay was attending elementary school and playing soccer. I was coaching Clay's team. I was also a committee chairperson for the Parent Teacher Organization (PTO) at each of my sons' schools. I was busy. Time passed.

October came. I still had the pain in my left breast area. Sometimes it hurt worse than other times. I tried to look for a pattern—maybe it was the weather, my extra weight—but I couldn't find one. I continued to manually check for lumps but could not find anything. I decided to try a new bra. That didn't work. I continued doing my manual breast exams but I still didn't feel anything out of the ordinary.

Finally, in late October, I decided to do a manual breast exam standing up. I let the weight of the breast rest on my cupped fingers and manipulated the area, again searching for anything. I paused. I felt something. I felt it for what seemed like an eternity. I stopped and re-positioned my fingers and palpated the area again. I felt it again. OK. *There is something there. I can feel it,* I thought. Of course, my mind started traveling in the wrong direction. But I quickly stopped those negative thoughts. Many women find lots of lumps and most are benign, I rationalized.

For the next several days, I checked the area. I waited for my monthly menstrual cycle to pass to see if the lump would disappear, as they sometimes do. After all, one of the things I'd learned this year was not to schedule a mammogram within the 10-day period after my menstrual cycle. I'd had a false reading on my mammogram in January 2008 for this reason. As a result, I had to have a magnetic resonance image (MRI). The MRI was negative, and the follow-up mammogram in February was also negative.

But the small lump was still there. Nevertheless, I told myself there was still no need to panic. After all, the MRI in January and the second mammogram in February had been negative. But the feeling that I needed to have it checked would not go away.

The holidays were approaching and I knew I would be busy. I was due for my annual gynecological exam in early December and for a mammogram in early January 2009. I rationalized: By the time I contacted my doctor and scheduled an appointment, it would be close to the date of my originally scheduled appointment anyway. So I waited. In the meantime, I would watch the area closely and see if the lump changed.

Something deep inside me told me that this was not an ordinary lump. However, I did what a lot of women do. I denied the lump's existence and dismissed the idea that it was anything more than a benign mass.

November came and I turned 49 years old. We celebrated Thanksgiving and prepared for the Christmas holidays. I remember being extremely tired. In early

December, I went for my gynecological exam and told the doctor about the lump. The doctor scheduled a mammogram and MRI for the first week in January 2009. Christmas came and we celebrated the season, taking our annual family portrait around the Christmas tree. After the portrait was taken, I looked at the picture. It was a portrait of my left side. I immediately felt as if the picture was nagging at me. Again, I could not break free of this worry. My thoughts turned to my upcoming mammogram. I needed to get past this mammogram to quiet my thoughts and fears. But somehow my women's intuition told me, the fear was not going to be laid to rest.

3

SNOW DAY

The holidays ended and January 2009 arrived. My children returned to school from Winter Break. My mammogram was scheduled the first week of the New Year.

The afternoon before, the weather started to deteriorate. An ice storm was making its way towards our area. The meteorologists were already announcing an ice advisory for the next day—the day I was scheduled to have my long-awaited mammogram.

I received a phone call from the breast center to remind me about my mammogram. The receptionist stated that I could keep the mammogram appointment or reschedule for a later date if the weather was bad. "We will be here anyway," she said, "but don't put yourself in any danger trying to make it to the scheduled appointment." OK, I thought. *I can cancel this appointment and put it off for a few more days.* When I look back, I realize I was in denial.

The next morning, most of the ice storm went south and the schools were on a two-hour delay. The streets were only lightly covered with snow. Even though I loved the thrill of driving in snowy weather, I was talking myself out of keeping my scheduled mammogram appointment. I did not want to face what I felt might be coming. Although I knew something was not right with this lump, I convinced myself to reschedule the appointment.

I put my sons on the school bus and made my way into the house to call to reschedule. It suddenly occurred to me that I was acting fearfully. I could not believe I was avoiding this again. *It's time for my yearly mammogram, for God's sake! It's my responsibility to do this for my family, let alone for myself!* So many times I had read about people putting off the inevitable, and here I was doing the same thing. This was so not me. Usually, I want to know results, and here I was avoiding the situation. How ridiculous that I thought the lump was going to take care of itself!

I quickly dressed and headed to my scheduled mammogram appointment. I arrived a few minutes late due to the slick highways. I could not delay this scan anymore. Besides, if my mammogram was clear, I was only dragging out the anxiety for no apparent reason. It was time to act. Finally, the nurse called my name. I followed her to the examination room for my mammogram. *__March Forth__* Marci, *__March Forth!__*

4
DIAGNOSIS

I walked down the hall to the examination room, realizing my stomach had butterflies. I had never felt that way before a mammogram. As the nurse prepared me for my scan, I thought about the mammogram jokes I'd received via e-mail. Every time one of my breasts is placed in the scanning machine, I think about those jokes. Humor has always helped me through stressful situations. Some of them are actually quite funny. I liked the jokes that advise women to prepare for mammograms by doing some exercises—for example, inserting your breast in an open doorway and slamming the door shut. Actually, inserting your breast in a freezer door would better prepare you for an actual mammogram because it would allow the breast to feel the full effect: a cold, compressed feeling much like the compression of the mammography machine itself.

I personally do not find mammograms that painful. However, if you think they are, then you are in pain for approximately 30 to 60 seconds.

I believe most women avoid mammograms because they are an inconvenience. I also believe women avoid them because they cannot afford them or want to avoid the fear that surrounds getting a mammogram—fear of the machine, fear of possible pain from the machine, and fear of finding a lump. (Contact the local American Cancer Society at www.cancer.org or the Susan G. Komen Foundation at www.komen.org for information about these issues.)

As the technician prepped me for my mammogram, she asked me the routine questions. She verified my name and asked me if I had any problems. (Gee! Here was the question I'd dreaded. My standard answer has always been "No, but I am concerned because my mother died from breast cancer.") This time I stated, "Yes, I am concerned about a small lump I found in my left breast." She stated she would scrutinize the area.

After taking the "pancake press" on each one of my breasts, I waited for the technician to review the images. When she returned, she stated that she did indeed see something suspicious in the left breast. She needed to take another image. She took another "pancake press" and left the room again. I sat in the chair waiting. Time was starting to stand still. I did not cry. I did not panic. I sat and stared. *My intuition had been right,* I thought. I'd known something wasn't right. I had hoped I was wrong, but my instincts had been correct all along. For the past four months, I realized, I'd been subconsciously building my mental strength. The technician returned. "We need to look at this further," she said. "Something does look suspicious. We have scheduled an ultrasound for further review." Though she told me that sometimes benign lumps look unusual, the suspicious area in my left breast needed further evaluation.

I was quickly moved to the ultrasound waiting room. My thoughts started cycling. My head was starting to hurt from the many thoughts crashing through it. Although most lumps are benign, I knew this lump was not. However, I would wait for the health professionals to confirm my suspicions.

My name was called for the ultrasound. I felt confident in the health professionals handling the procedure. As the ultrasound was administered, both the radiologist and ultrasound technician saw something that looked suspicious in my left breast. Neither one would validate that it was definitely breast cancer; only a biopsy could confirm that. However, both professionals all but stated it *was* breast cancer. My thoughts raced faster as I faced the reality that I had breast cancer. Nevertheless, I would have to wait for the biopsy for official confirmation.

Thus, the ultrasound confirmed what the mammogram had shown. Something was abnormal. A biopsy was scheduled. However, the first available biopsy appointment was next week. I would have to wait *nine days* before I would know definitely if the lump was breast cancer!

The ultrasound technician was empathetic. She disliked the fact I had to wait more than a week to confirm the diagnosis. She stated that the breast center would call me if a biopsy appointment became available sooner due to a cancellation. "Be ready for the call because it may be as little as an hour before the scheduled time of the biopsy!" she said.

Again, I did not panic. I did not cry. I dressed and walked to my car to go home. My brain was numb. When I look back at this moment, I realize I was in shock. I thought I had been handed a death sentence. After seeing what my mother had been through, I was now walking in her shoes. I was facing something I had hoped I would never have to face again, especially after seeing Mom and my father-in-law die in the last four years from this dreaded disease.

5

"IT IS WHAT IT IS"

January 2008 verses January 2009

Driving home, I was still very calm. I still did not cry. I was numb. I was in shock. This was totally opposite from what I had been like a year ago. In January 2008, the breast center had called to tell me my mammogram was abnormal and I needed an MRI and a follow-up mammogram. I'd cried uncontrollably as I called Steve at work. Steve tried to calm me on the phone. "We will get through this—just like we did with Clay," he said.

Clay's Birth

Two years after Corey's birth and before Clay was born, I had a miscarriage. I was in the doctor's office waiting for my appointment with my mother. It was the first and only office visit she came to with me during my three pregnancies. I was glad she was there. It was my three-month visit and it was the day I was going to hear the baby's heartbeat for the first time.

But things started unraveling during my examination. They could not find the heartbeat. As the appointment progressed, it became apparent that there was no heartbeat and the fetus had died. It was one of the most heart-wrenching things I had ever experienced. (I believe miscarriage is much harder on the mother than the father because you already have a bond with the child you are carrying. I feel fathers do not get to experience that type of bond until the baby is born.)

My husband, my minister, and my boss helped me through this crisis. What seemed like an eternity at that moment was really a short span of time. Life continued, and six months later I was pregnant again, with Clay. I was nervous and reserved during that pregnancy. A lot of people choose not to tell friends and family about their pregnancies until they are several months along, especially after losing one to miscarriage. But, I didn't feel that way. I had another living child growing inside of me! I had to validate that this child existed even if I might lose this one to miscarriage, too. Steve and I approached this pregnancy cautiously. I knew this would be the last time I would try for a child because I was 38 years old. Only time would tell if this child would make it.

I was approximately seven weeks into my pregnancy when I was rushed to the hospital. I had started hemorrhaging. I was crying uncontrollably because I knew I was losing this child, too. The faces of the emergency room doctor and nurse looked grim. They could not find a fetal heartbeat. A gynecologist was called into the emergency room. He took me to another department for an ultrasound to determine whether there was a viable fetus. Lo and behold, the doctor found a heartbeat! It was beating at 80 beats per minute. "Miscarriage is 60 heartbeats," he said. "The fetus needs to be around 120 heartbeats. But, we still have a baby!" He put me on bed rest and told me to return three days later for another heartbeat check. The next three days were critical if the fetus was going to make it. The seconds went by excruciatingly slowly each day. When we returned to the doctor's office, the baby's heartbeat was back to 120 beats. It was only the beginning of a roller-coaster ride for us and for this baby over the next six months.

After seven months of bed rest, a trip to the hospital to stop labor, and weekly visits to the doctor, my gynecologist made an important discovery. He checked the amniotic fluid levels in my placenta at 7½ months and found there was hardly any. The placenta was dying and would not support the fetus anymore. We had to start labor if the baby was going to survive. Labor was induced, and Clay was born. He was immediately rushed to the Intensive Care Unit and put on life support. After two exhaustive weeks in the ICU, our little Clay _Marched Forth_ and came home a healthy six-pound boy.

But this crisis was different, I tried to tell Steve. This diagnosis was about my life or death. I was panicked. He tried to calm me on the phone. Thank God the mammogram and MRI were negative on my follow-up visits in

February 2008.

Now, however—one year later—I was *almost certain* something was wrong. The ultrasound and mammogram were confirming my suspicions. As I drove home, I felt dazed. Suddenly, nothing seemed to matter. All the little things such as laundry, errands, and housework vanished. I thought about my kids. My biggest fear was coming true: My fear of dying before they were old enough to take care of themselves was staring me in the face. God knew this fear of mine. I had talked to Him about it.

I called my husband at work. I had tried to prepare him that morning before I went for my mammogram. "Something is wrong!" I'd told him. I don't think he took me seriously because of the false-positive results a year earlier. But now I was calling to inform him that they did indeed see something suspicious and I needed to pursue it further. "The mammogram and ultrasound found some questionable areas," I said. "I have to have a biopsy!" Steve tried to reassure me just like he had a year ago. But now I was trying to prepare him for the worst news. "The ultrasound _was_ indicating lobular breast cancer," I said. "However, it cannot be confirmed until the biopsy is performed and the tissue tested." Although he was trying to stay positive, I was trying to convince him of a harsh reality. "Most likely, this will not be a false diagnosis like last year," I said. "These were health professionals who were experienced in pinpointing this disease during mammograms and ultrasounds." I relayed the information about waiting until next week for the biopsy.

Steve and I would have to wait patiently several days for a confirmation to determine whether or not the mass was breast cancer.

Waiting was a killer. If there was a tumor in my breast, I wanted it out immediately. I did not want it growing any more or staying inside me any longer. I felt as if I had a time bomb inside of me. I wanted it dealt with as soon as possible. But now I was facing a whole week before I could have a biopsy! In all probability, it would be two full weeks of waiting to confirm that I had cancer growing inside my breast!

As I left the breast center, I was given lots of literature about breast cancer. When I arrived home, I set the literature aside. I was too overwhelmed to read it. It would not sink into my mind that I had breast cancer.

Two days passed. Luck was on my side. The breast center called. Someone had cancelled their appointment and they had an opening for a biopsy. The nurse asked, "Can you get here in 40 minutes?" "Yes!" I said. I called Steve. He left work and met me at the breast center.

A biopsy was taken from two spots: the left breast and the right breast. The biopsy was not painful, but I did feel a slight pinch. The spot in the right breast did not appear nearly as suspicious as the spot taken in the left breast. But nonetheless, a sample was taken as a precautionary measure. Again, the physician and technician were quite concerned about the suspicious area in the left breast. The technician repeatedly asked me if I was OK. I reassured her I was. I tried to remain upbeat during the procedure but I felt very dull and heavy inside.

She commented on how strong I was being and that a lot of patients start crying or breaking down at this point. She was concerned for my mental state. I said, "Thanks, but it is what it is and nothing I can do right now is going to change what is there." Again, these professionals were most certain it was breast cancer but needed to wait for the biopsy results to officially confirm the diagnosis.

After the biopsy, I left the doctor's office to drive home. Again, everything seemed surreal. I was doing better, but I was still in shock. I couldn't cry or react or do much of anything. I was floating mentally as I descended from the fifth floor of the parking garage in my car. My world was quiet. It felt as if everything had stopped around me. My time stood still. These medical professionals were telling me I most likely had breast cancer, I repeatedly told myself! It would not sink in! *I am too young to have breast cancer!*

How could I have cancer? I'd just turned 49 in November. I ate healthy food. I didn't have high blood pressure or high cholesterol. I maintained my weight. I walked, did yoga, and lifted weights. *I have high HDL! That was a good thing, damn it!* However, I realized none of these entitled me to a long life. Maybe stress was the culprit. God knows what we had been through in the last few years. Was it the strain of all the illnesses, deaths, and work? But didn't the healthy eating and exercising eliminate the stresses?! *Wow!* was all I could think. I talked to God. *We will get through this,* I thought. I prayed that I would see my kids grow up into young, healthy men. They were my first thoughts. I wanted to experience all of the important milestones in their life. *Am I going to be there for them? Will I see their graduations, marriages, and my possible grandchildren? Steve will be OK,* I thought. At least my sons were old enough to help themselves at ages 10 and 13 years.

I continued to drive on the expressway towards home. I was in shock and deep in thought. When I arrived home, I thought, *whom do I call? Whom do I let know? Do I keep it quiet? When do I tell my kids? How do I explain this when I cannot comprehend it myself?* I decided to wait until the biopsy results were confirmed.

After a nightmarish week of mammograms, ultrasounds, and biopsies, the breast center finally called to relay the results. "The biopsy confirms that you have infiltrating (invasive) lobular breast cancer," the nurse said. Although I already knew in my heart that I had cancer, hearing the nurse tell me was overwhelming and shocking. After talking with the nurse briefly about the results, I hung up. I began my prayers. I asked God to give me strength and help me **_March Forth_** through this challenge that awaited my family and me.

6
DECISIONS, DECISIONS

Wow! I sat on my bed. *Now what?* I knew *I* had to handle this news first before I could tell anyone else in my family. Once I broke the news to them, I would become their comforter. I had to be strong for them as well as for myself. What an exhausting thought that was in itself! I knew Steve would be my rock when I told him. He would be strong support as he has always been through all of our previous challenges. But how do I tell the others. *How do I tell my kids*, who had lost their grandmother and grandfather to cancer? *How do I tell my sister and my brothers? Oh my God, how do I tell my dad*, who was married to Mom for 58 years and lost her to breast cancer, that his daughter now has breast cancer? *Am I going to die from this, too?* What a horrific struggle my mom and father-in-law went through before they died. *Am I going to struggle as well?* My mind was racing. I had to call my husband and tell him the results. What a lonely feeling it was to sit on the edge of my bed and try to digest this information. After collecting myself somewhat, I called Steve.

"The results are back from my biopsies," I said. "I

have infiltrating lobular breast cancer." Wow! Just saying those words made me feel detached. *It just cannot be true,* I thought. I was choking on the words as I spoke. "They have a packet of information for me at the main desk at the breast center," I said. "Can you please pick this information up for me on your way home from work?" Even though Steve and I knew the results of the biopsy was most likely cancer, the reality of hearing I had breast cancer hit us hard.

I hung up the phone and lay down on the bed. I was already mentally exhausted from the previous week's roller-coaster ride. This news made me want to collapse. I wanted to lie down and sleep. Maybe, after a nap, I would wake up and this would all be a bad dream. I was suddenly overwhelmed with what seemed like a thousand questions that needed answers and a thousand decisions I needed to make. I had no idea where I was going, but I knew I had to *__March Forth__* with all my strength. I lay down to take a nap and wait for my children to come home from school on the bus.

7

A LIFE-CHANGING EVENT

An hour later my kids bounced through the door, home from school. Corey, my quiet, internal son, and Clay, my outward, social son, were creatures of habit. This afternoon was no different for them than any other—turn on the TV, grab a snack, and answer a "Hey, how was your day?" I looked at them, admiring their free spirits. Their energy was uplifting. However, I knew I would soon put a damper on their spirits because of the results that I'd found out that day.

Neither son had a clue as to what I had been going through the past week. I had not told them about my appointments and had hidden my emotions to shield them from this shocking news. I knew it would be devastating to them because they had lost two grandparents to cancer. They'd seen firsthand what cancer can do to a person. I worried about how to tell them. I decided I would wait for the weekend to break the news. I kept the results to myself and went about my business as if nothing were wrong.

I had several reasons why I chose not to tell our children immediately about my results. I did not want them to be distracted from their schoolwork. Besides, the weekend would give them more opportunities to digest the news and ask questions before they would have to go back to school. Maybe it would also give me time to accept it as well. I could think of lots of excuses why not to tell them. It was another way I could deny the cancer's existence. But no matter how many excuses I could think of for not telling our children that I had breast cancer, the biggest excuse was the worst. I was going to hurt my children when I told them the news. As a parent and mother, I hated that.

It is a challenging event to tell your children news that you know will hurt them. As their mother, it's my responsibility to protect them from the hurts of the world. I knew the news would hurt them. They had experienced cancer firsthand with their grandmother and grandfather. I remembered the bedtime discussion I'd had with my children when Mom was about to pass. I tried to explain that Grandma was very, very sick. Corey began to understand. He asked, "Mommy is Grandma going to die?" I hesitated and searched for the proper answer. I had to tell them both the truth. "Yes, Grandma is going to die," I said. It hurt me to say it and feel it. But it hurt me worse to tell my children they were going to lose their grandma.

Again, I faced confronting my children with hurtful news. Hopefully, I could digest the information myself and prepare to tell them later. After a few days, it became apparent I would have to tell them sooner than planned. I was getting messages on my answering machine from the breast center about setting up different tests and doctors' appointments. I did not want my kids to find out from another source, so I realized I could not put it off any longer.

I will not forget the looks on their faces when I told them I had breast cancer. They knew the potential consequences. I told them I was confident we had caught the breast cancer early and my chances of survival were very good. Although the prognosis was good, I knew I could not guarantee them 100 percent that I was going to be OK. My job was to reassure them that I felt confident in my doctors and test results and that I would get the best care. I told them the next few months were going to be very challenging for all of us and we would all need to do our best at school and at home. All of us would need to **_March Forth_** with all our strength and prayers.

8

... AND MORE DECISIONS!

After telling our children the news, I began digesting the fact that I had breast cancer. I was inundated with decisions and appointments. I skimmed the Internet for information. There was a lot of material on the Internet but some of it was confusing and contradictory. I decided I was going to limit myself to three to four well-known websites and make my final decisions.

First I had to schedule several tests. I had to schedule and complete a breast MRI so the surgeon could pinpoint the tumor. I had to have a bone scan to determine if the cancer had spread to my bones. I had to give blood samples for analysis. I had to give more blood samples for more analysis. I continued to give more blood samples for more analysis until I thought I would need a transfusion. (I began to hate the needle pricks.)

I had to choose a surgeon and then schedule a consultation. I had to determine if I wanted a lumpectomy, mastectomy, or double mastectomy. If I wanted the lumpectomy, did I want the cell-enhanced breast reconstruction (fat graft) or the quadrantectomy with breast reduction for symmetry? What type of mastectomy did I need? Did I need a simple/total, modified radical, radical/Halsted, or skin-sparing mastectomy? Did I want reconstruction of my breast? If I chose reconstruction, what type of reconstruction did I want? Did I want implanted reconstruction or autologous reconstruction? If I did decide on implant reconstruction, did I want saline or silicone? If I decided to have autologous reconstruction, did I want the skin and tummy fat microsurgery or the skin and buttock microsurgery? If I chose the tummy fat microsurgery, did I want the DIEP flap or the SIEA flap? If I chose the skin and buttock microsurgery, did I want the IGAP flap or SGAP flap?[1] Good heavens! It was overwhelming trying to decide what I wanted. (Jeez! It was like ordering a hamburger at a fast-food restaurant. Did I want ketchup, mustard, mayonnaise, or salad dressing? Did I want American, Swiss, or Colby cheese? Did I want lettuce, pickle, relish, or all the above?) The more I read, the more confused I became. The information was overwhelming and I was already on overload trying to accept the fact that I had breast cancer. However, my main concern at this point was getting the damn tumor out!

It was overwhelming. I'd gone from being a healthy individual to one who suddenly was very sick. Mentally and physically, I still felt healthy. I started hating the hospitals and doctors' offices because they were making me feel sicker than I thought I was. Going through this process can really overwhelm your psyche. However, I was trying not to let the negativity dictate my well-being. *I am not as sick as they think,* I told myself.

If I ever needed a sign to reinforce that thought, it

came the next day as I was cleaning out my laundry room. (Cleaning was keeping my mind occupied and helping me to digest my diagnosis.) I found a present that I had wrapped an amazing 25 years ago. I was planning to give it to a friend, but she'd left town and I'd never given it to her. I had forgotten that I had stored the present on a shelf in my laundry room. I knew it was a book but had forgotten which one. I opened the present.

The book was *You Can't Afford the Luxury of a Negative Thought: A Book for People with Any Life—Threatening Illness-Including Life,* by John-Rodgers and Peter McWilliams. It described how positive thoughts produce positive results.

Wow, I thought. When I read the title of the book again, I stopped dead in my tracks. Was this another coincidence? I immediately went upstairs and began reading the book.

I realized I was feeling several negative thoughts. I was downbeat and depressed. I was in denial and pessimistic. My body was tense and filled with anxiety. I was very fatigued from worry. I realized I needed to focus on changing my negative thoughts to positive thoughts so I could produce positive results. My negative thoughts were not helping my cause. I put the book on the table by my bed. Each night the book reminded me to focus on positive thoughts to produce positive results.

Thus, I changed my attitude. I focused on having happy, optimistic, upbeat, and encouraging thoughts. Positive thoughts would allow me to feel better and be more productive. It was hard at first to catch and change my negative thoughts into positive thoughts, but I knew I had to do it. I couldn't control the cancer, but I could control my attitude. I prayed for strength, encouragement, and healing. I asked God to help me and remind me to positively ___*March Forth!*___

9
FACT VERSES FICTION

One of the most frustrating things I encountered through the whole diagnosis process was the waiting. Shortly after the breast center informed me I had infiltrating lobular breast cancer (ILC), I was scheduled for a consultation with the surgeon—10 days later! I wanted to meet with him *tomorrow!* This was an emergency! I had a cancerous tumor growing inside of me, for heaven's sake! Thus, for 10 days, I tried my darnedest to find all the information I could about ILC. I needed to know everything I could before making a decision. Thank goodness for the Internet (I think?)! I started reading everything about breast cancer. I became familiar with the terminology so I could ask informed questions of my surgeon and oncologist. Sometimes, late at night, I would get out of bed and read because I couldn't sleep. I searched for facts and tried to foresee the possible scenarios. Sometimes the information was scary and sometimes it was informative; however, I wanted to know. Here are a few facts that I found out about breast cancer:

- Infiltrating (Invasive) lobular breast (ILC) cancer is the second most commonly diagnosed breast cancer. Approximately 10 percent of breast cancers are diagnosed as ILC. (*Lobular* refers to the lobules where milk is produced.)[2]
- Invasive ductal breast cancer (IDC) is the most commonly diagnosed breast cancer. Approximately 80 percent of breast cancers are diagnosed as IDC. (*Ductal* refers to the ducts where the milk flows from the lobules.)[3]
- Approximately 10 percent of breast cancers are diagnosed as rare or uncommon breast cancers.[4]
- Men can get breast cancer. Fewer than 1 percent of all breast cancers occur in men.[5]
- Two-thirds of women are 55 years of age or older when diagnosed with invasive breast cancer. However, breast cancer can occur at any age.[6]
- ILC has a tendency to occur in women in their early sixties. (Why was I diagnosed so young, at age 49?)[7]
- IDC has a tendency to occur in women in their middle fifties.[8]
- IDC usually forms a lump. ILC usually forms a spiraling, long, irregular border. Thus, ILC is harder to image. It also is tougher to get a clear margin with ILC than IDC because of its irregular border. The average diameter of ILC when found is about 2 to 5 centimeters. (I felt very fortunate my two tumors were only 0.5 and 0.6 centimeters.)[9]
- ILC has a higher reoccurrence rate in the second

breast than IDC.[10]

- The risk of metastasis is relatively low if the diagnosis (of the cancer stage) is found early.[11]
- The earlier the cancer stage is found, the greater the survival rate.[12]

10

THE SURGEON'S VISIT

After two weeks of waiting and scanning the Internet, the day to visit my surgeon finally arrived on January 22, 2009. It was great to actually proceed forward with some type of positive action towards removing the cancer in my breast. It did wonders for my psyche.

The surgeon and I discussed the pathology report from my breast biopsies. The right breast biopsy was benign and the left breast biopsy revealed two infiltrating lobular breast tumors of five and six millimeters each. The hormone receptors of the tumors indicated I had estrogen-receptor-positive (ER-positive) breast cancer (estrogen 83% and progesterone 8%). This was a good thing. The higher the breast tissue tested positive to the estrogen receptors, the better were my chances of treating the disease. I was informed that the cure rate was at least 95 percent if there was no lymph node involvement. There was an extremely good chance of no lymph node involvement because my tumors were small; however, we would have to wait until the lymph nodes were tested during surgery before we knew for sure. We had caught the cancer early due to my yearly exams and the great medical employees who had successfully done their jobs.

The surgeon and I discussed several options. Treatment could range from a lumpectomy and possible radiation to a double mastectomy. After further discussion, we decided it would be beneficial for me to take the genetic tests called the BRCA1/BRCA2 (tests that look for the breast and ovarian cancer susceptibility genes). The genetic tests would help me decide whether to follow a mild or aggressive treatment plan to eliminate the cancer. We would make a decision based on the results.

Thus, I left the surgeon's office and went to the lab to have blood drawn for the BRCA1/BRCA2 tests. I would have to wait two to six weeks for the test results to come back before I could finalize an action plan. In the meantime, I was scheduled for a bone scan on January 26, 2009, to evaluate the pain in my left rib area. I marched out of the doctor's office with a partial action plan. However, I did not have enough answers at this point to reduce my anxiety, which continued to build because I was again waiting for results.

The BRCA1/BRCA2 tests were fairly new tests. It made sense for me to take them since my family had a strong history of breast cancer. The only problem with this course of action was that my blood samples had to be sent to a lab located several states away—hence the additional two to six week wait for the results! There were reasons why it would take so long. One, only a few labs in the United States could perform these tests. Two, the insurance companies required a lot of paperwork, and processing this paperwork took a lot of time.

Three, many insurance companies deny the tests because of their cost or don't cover them because they are considered out of the ordinary tests. (Ahhh! The Great Paper Trail at its best!) These tests had only become available locally in the last two to three years. In fact, when I went to have my blood drawn for the tests, it was the first time the technician had ever taken a blood sample for the BRCA1/BRCA2 tests.

The surgeon's office informed us that these tests may be denied by the insurance company because of the expense or exempted under a clause in the insurance policy. The tests themselves cost approximately $4,000. We would have to pay it out of our pockets if the insurance denied it. Steve and I proceeded with the tests. The last thing we wanted to do was play Russian roulette with my life. If these BRCA1/BRCA2 genetic tests came back positive, it meant I had an _extremely high chance_ of developing cancer in my other breast and/or my ovaries.

After giving the blood sample, I went home. Four days later, I went for my bone scan. I was having pain in my rib area near the breast that contained the tumors. Although the surgeon didn't think I had cancer in the rib area, we did the bone scan as a precaution. My bone scan was negative.

After the bone scan, I called the breast center and requested to see an oncologist (a cancer specialist) but was advised to wait and schedule a visit _after_ my surgery. However, the information I read on the Internet encouraged me to see an oncologist _before_ my surgery. Thus, I called the breast center back and insisted on an appointment with an oncologist. It was scheduled for February 2, 2009. Again, it was time for me to sit back and wait. Things were progressing, but not nearly as fast as I wished they would. All I could do was keep my attitude positive and *__March Forth.__*

11

"I HAVE BREAST CANCER"

Girlfriends Needed . . . My Final Decision

Finally, February 2009 arrived. I was glad to put January behind me. It had been a roller-coaster ride all month.

February meant going forward in a positive direction, I told myself. Things were finally starting to move—or so I thought. I called my family and told them: "I have breast cancer." I told my girlfriends as I ran into them: "I have breast cancer!" Each time I said it, it made me face and validate the fact: *I have breast cancer!*

The reality of what I was facing was staring at me point-blank. One minute I was trying to reassure myself everything was going to be alright and then the next I was crying and disillusioned, convinced that I was going to die. The fact that I had breast cancer brought indescribable shock and thoughts. It was still hard for me to believe because I thought I was young, healthy, and athletic. But I needed to deal with it. Unfortunately, the cards had been dealt, and I'd gotten the two of spades.

For now, it was time to find solutions and "fix it." It was time to realize the death of my breast was coming and I had to prepare myself to handle this journey physically and emotionally.

One day while I was still waiting for my test results, my thoughts started churning in the wrong direction. I called my good friend Carolyn (an angel) who worked in the health field. "What does this phrase mean in my pathology report?" I asked. I had been studying my biopsy results that afternoon, hoping to understand some of the terminology. It began backfiring on me. Suddenly, I was reading more into the report than I should have. I thought my doctor was not telling me everything I needed to know. I was also starting to understand the reality of my situation and felt like I was going to die. I started to panic. I started crying. She quickly came over to my home and calmed my fears. She reassured me that everything was going to be OK—words I needed to hear at that moment and would need to hear often over the next several months. You can never hear that enough throughout this process. "You are going to be OK!" It was overwhelming, to say the least. As I said before, sometimes you can read too much information and sometimes it's best to leave it alone. (Everyone has to find that balance for herself when she faces this situation.)

Of course, everyone had an idea as to what I should do. I was willing to listen to all their thoughts. I was not offended. I wanted to know if there was something I was not seeing or thinking through completely. Their ideas ranged from removing both breasts immediately to having a simple lumpectomy. Some definitely would have reconstruction, others would not. The responses included "You are finished using your breasts," "Your children have grown and your breasts are not needed any more," "Breasts are the symbol of being a woman." "It would be a no-brainer to have reconstruction," and so on." Wow! I really had to laugh at some of the responses!

But all humor and emotions aside, I did have to make a decision. After talking with my doctor, reading many articles, and searching the Internet, I came to a conclusion. Each woman has to make this decision on her own. It is her body and she has to live with it. She has to be comfortable with what she has chosen and what she will look like after the decision. For me, reconstruction was about taking on a part of me that was not real. No matter how I tried to hide or fix this situation, it was not going to be the God- given breast I'd had before this nightmare began. It was the death of my breast. I could not bring it back to life. I would chalk it up as one of life's cruelties.

Thus, I decided to make it simple. After all, it was not about replacing my breast. It was about ridding my body of the cancer. I selected a unilateral (one-sided) mastectomy with no reconstruction. I would be fitted with a prosthesis after surgery. That was all I could handle at that point in my treatment. I couldn't speculate about what might happen in the future but only decide what I needed to do right then. I told myself I could leave my options open, saving a possible reconstruction or mastectomy of the other breast for the future. But for now, I wanted to focus on what I needed first and foremost—to get through this initial crisis. A unilateral mastectomy with no reconstruction was my final answer unless the BRCA1/BRCA2 test results affected this decision. Now I could begin to _**March Forth**_ towards eradicating this disease from my body.

12

MY FINAL DECISION

During the process of reaching my final decision to have a mastectomy, I studied many possible treatments. First, the most conservative choice was a lumpectomy (excising the lump or tumor). My surgeon stated that a lumpectomy with possible radiation treatments was standard protocol for my diagnosis. I did not want to have radiation, due to the side effects. If I had the mastectomy, most likely I would not need to have radiation because the tumors were small.

If I had chosen a lumpectomy, I would have to make sure the excised area had a clear margin, (that cancerous breast tissue was surrounded by healthy tissue when removed). If the cancerous tissue did not have a clear margin, then I would need to return for more surgery to remove more tissue or possibly the whole breast. I wanted to get it right the first time. I did not want to go back for more surgery and anesthesia.

Also, if I had chosen a lumpectomy, the affected breast would be smaller than my other breast. I would still have to wear a partial prosthesis or undergo some type of reconstruction to make it match my other breast. I felt it would be easier to remove my whole breast and match the remaining breast. Either way, it was very important to have an excellent plastic surgeon for any type of reconstruction.

If I had chosen a mastectomy with implant reconstruction, it would have been an immediate fix. But I took a long-term view. I would love my body to stay young, but life proceeds ahead. Unfortunately, as women age, life's natural processes do take place: gravity, menopause, and weight gain/loss. Each would affect the shape of my natural breast over time. But, the reconstructed breast would not be affected. The implant would not change in shape or diameter. This would be great if I were replacing both breasts. However, since I was only removing one breast, it could create the problem of possibly having a lopsided appearance. In other words, my God-given breast would begin to sag and change as I aged and the other breast would forever remain twenty-something.

If I had chosen reconstruction and an implant, I knew I did not want to undergo the process of expanders. (This process stretches skin and muscles before inserting the implant.) I would also need to replace the implant after several years. I did not want to face more surgery and anesthesia when I was 60 or 70 years old or if something happened to the implants while they were in my body.

Also, reconstruction requires more surgery and anesthesia. I did not want more surgery and anesthesia.

More surgery would increase my chances of infection, especially staph infection. I read some horror stories about women who tried unsuccessfully to have implant surgery only to find they were wearing a breast prosthesis in the end. I did not want to increase my chances of fighting this infection while healing from a mastectomy. Furthermore, *if* I had to have chemotherapy and/or radiation after the surgery, it would have been overwhelming to handle the mastectomy, chemotherapy, radiation, possible staph infection, and the process of stretching the breast area to prepare for an implant.

If I had to choose a type of reconstruction, I would select the autologous reconstruction. This reconstruction would use my own body fat to reconstruct my breast. Depending on the area of my body I selected, I could have the extra benefit of a tummy tuck or buttocks tuck. (These are the most popular areas from which to take fat for this surgery.) The disadvantage of autologous reconstruction was that I would have another surgical area that needed to heal and another site for a possible staph infection in addition to the mastectomy surgical site. However, I liked the thought of having my own parts rather than a foreign object in my body.

All of these choices were overwhelming me. Therefore, I kept it simple. For now I was going to have a unilateral mastectomy. I wanted to concentrate on freeing myself of cancer, not making myself prettier. What good would it do to be prettier, when I felt as if I were going to die anyway? (That thought kept rearing its ugly head!) I was not thinking straight, and I didn't want to make a decision I'd regret later. Thus, for now, I would tackle just the mastectomy.

After I made my decision, I found that many in the medical field assumed I would want reconstruction after my mastectomy. In fact, I felt some pressure to choose reconstruction and felt odd for not wanting it. (Sometimes I thought the medical field was preying on women's emotions. Reconstruction is definitely a moneymaker for some doctors.)

It's important to do the research and make sure your choice is right for you. It was a hard decision for me because I was still trying to digest my diagnosis and make logical decisions about my health care. I tried to keep everything in perspective. After all, we were talking about life versus aesthetics. What is more important here?

I admire women who make the choice to have reconstruction. If that is what they want and it makes them feel whole again, so be it. And it is easier nowadays to have reconstruction following a mastectomy. Many mastectomies and reconstruction surgeries are scheduled back to back, making it easier on patients since they have two surgeries scheduled under one anesthesia.

I decided against the double mastectomy because the other breast was "healthy." It was not diseased. Why would I remove something that was OK? I wanted to live for today, not for what might happen tomorrow. Besides, research was showing no difference in the survival rate of those women who opted for a mastectomy and those who chose a lumpectomy *for my diagnosis.* Furthermore, no treatment would provide me with the absolute guarantee that cancer would not return. If there were such a surefire treatment, every person diagnosed with breast cancer would be getting it!

Furthermore, scientists and researchers are making giant strides every day. New treatments are found to help breast cancer survival as I write. I wanted to see my glass as half full, not half empty. My sister Michele was especially concerned with my choice. She did not want me to have to go through the same pain my mom had. "I read and researched this thoroughly and I feel comfortable with my decision," I told her. "Besides, let's give the breast cancer a target in my good breast *if* it dares to come back," I joked. Losing one breast was traumatic enough. At this point, I just couldn't mentally handle losing both breasts, especially my healthy one.

Another reason I chose a unilateral mastectomy was because of the type of breast cancer I had been diagnosed with. Lobular cancer is often labeled "sneaky." It grows in a line more so than a lump, spiraling out like a web. This makes it harder to see on a mammogram until it is very large. What if there were more spots in the breast but technology could not see them? My breasts were extremely dense, which makes it harder to see irregularities on a mammogram. Thus, my diagnosis was only as good as the medical technology and personnel executing and reading the tests.

Another reason I chose a unilateral mastectomy was that I wanted to focus on today, on now—not tomorrow! *Let me focus on what I need to deal with now. I only have today.* It's all any of us have.

After I made my final decision, I told Steve. Although he felt it was my decision, he was glad my final choice was a mastectomy without reconstruction. And even though it was my choice, I was relieved that he agreed with my decision. It helped me immensely that he supported my decision. (Attention, men! Please support your wives and girlfriends with their final decisions! Your support is very crucial during this process!)

Our society places so much emphasis on women's looks. I think this emphasis can create a lot of insecurity and ill-advised decisions for women trying to decide on their treatment. Even the strongest of women can feel fragile about their appearance. If I was ever going to "walk the walk," now was the time. I was always telling my children, "Beauty comes from the inside out—not the outside in." The beauty inside me would not change unless I mentally allowed it to. *Cancer cannot take my positive attitude,* I thought. *God will not take away the beauty He gave me inside.* Therefore, my decision was final. I would wait for the results of the BRCA1/BRCA2 tests. If they came back positive, it was a no-brainer to have the double mastectomy and oophorectomy (removal of the ovaries). But if they were negative, I would have a unilateral (one-sided) mastectomy. Another decision was made; it was time to ***March Forth.***

After I made my decision, I told Steve to be prepared for what I would look like without my breast. I explained to him that there would be a large scar. I suggested he look at a picture of a woman after a mastectomy on the Internet. I knew what to expect. My mom had undergone a double mastectomy. Maybe the way she'd handled her double mastectomy was helping me handle my unilateral mastectomy. Even though she was gone, she was still helping me to get through this journey. Again, I needed to ***March Forth.***

13

A FEW BUMPS IN THE ROAD

The Insurance Dilemma

Shortly after I was diagnosed with my breast cancer in January 2009, Steve came home from work and informed me that the small subsidiary company he worked for had been "let go" by its parent corporation. This meant our insurance was ending at the end of the month in 3 weeks. As a result, his company was searching for new insurance to cover its employees. We just looked at each other. We were not sure how this was going to affect my choice of hospitals, doctors, and—more importantly—my health coverage. The new insurance would take effect on February 1, 2009. Would they now exempt me because of my diagnosis? Would it be considered a preexisting condition? We were very nervous and concerned. We tried to stay upbeat and wait for the news. After all, it was going to be what it was going to be. Finally, our insurance was established and I was elated to find my current health care providers were available through our new health plan. No changes were necessary at this point.

The Oncology Visit

On February 2, 2009, I had my first oncology visit. I'd had to be insistent with the breast center to receive this appointment. I had asked to see my mother's oncologist. I'd thought highly of him when she was going through her treatment and thought I would feel comfortable having him for my medical treatment as well.

My visit was extremely upbeat and informative. My new doctor was very proactive towards my medical care. He immediately scheduled a CT/PET scan for my chest, abdominal cavity, and pelvis. He also scheduled an MRI for my brain. Though he felt the cancer was not in these areas, he wanted to complete the necessary tests as precautionary checks. It also gave us a baseline for future reference.

The oncologist felt we had caught the cancer early and my outlook was very good. I told him I was waiting for the results of my BRCA1/BRCA2 tests and was concerned about waiting all this time to do surgery. "I wanted to do something proactive," I said. "It has been five weeks and nothing has been done to prevent or stop the cancer!" The oncologist addressed my concerns immediately. He started me on a prescription drug to block my cells' receptors from receiving estrogen. Since my cancer tumors were estrogen-receptor positive, blocking the cells' receptors from receiving estrogen would cause the tumor to die or shrink.

Finally, we were progressing in the right direction. After my oncology visit, I felt better mentally. We were acting positively now to eradicate the cancer.

The Insurance Dilemma Again

On February 3, 2009, I spent my whole day on the phone trying to organize my upcoming scans and tests. This was hard to do without a proper insurance card. "I have insurance but my policy number has not been processed yet!" I pleaded. "I will have the card next week!" I knew I was fighting a losing battle here. How many people who actually did not have insurance requested health care and said that the card was in the mail so they could get treatment? I was a "broken record" to the billing department. Finally, I went ahead and scheduled the scans and tests and told them I would try to find out the policy number by the time I showed up for my appointments. (Some scans were scheduled for the next day.)

After scheduling my appointments, I called my husband's workplace and tried to connect with the representative for our new insurance. I explained what was happening, and both the insurance representative and Steve's work personnel tried to process the information as quickly as possible. But due to the time constraints, the insurance change happened at the worst possible time in my treatment process. Processing the paperwork would take time. (I applaud the efforts of those trying to get the policy number to me as quickly as possible.)

I called the breast center and informed them of my situation. I didn't know if I should reschedule my scans and tests for after I had the insurance card. They advised me not to reschedule but to move forward. I should not delay any longer. Thus, I proceeded with my appointments and waited for my policy number to arrive in the mail.

Arriving for my Appointments

On the morning of February 4, 2009, I began to prep myself for the tests and scans I had scheduled for that afternoon. The insurance card dilemma the previous day had been stressful. I was looking forward to this new day. I'd begun my fast the night before, then drank the "tasty liquid" at the appropriate times so I would "glow" for the tests. I was ready to go. Again, these tests were positive actions towards ridding the cancer from my body.

As I was preparing to leave, I saw the warmer weather had melted most of the snow, creating a glaze of ice on our sloping driveway. I backed out of my garage and stalled in the ice halfway up my driveway. *Great!* I thought. I drove the car back down the driveway and quickly sped up it again. (I only needed to drive another 20 feet or so to get to the highway!) I was stuck. I tried this several times. Each time I tried, I failed to get up the slight incline, and no one was around to help me push the car to freedom. I was getting angry. I had gotten out of my driveway all weekend in the snow, but the ice was a different story.

I turned my car around at the bottom of the driveway and tried again. I started digging and pouring sand around the tires, but I couldn't get the tires to grip. I soon realized I was not going to be able to dig my car out in time for the appointment at this rate. I started hauling hot water out of the house and melting the ice to gain traction. But again, this was not a fast fix, given how long my driveway was, and was not going to get me to my appointment on time.

I tried putting rugs under my wheels to give them traction. Again, no luck. The only thing this created was a comical scene of my rugs flying out from the back of my vehicle. They propelled like rockets every time I pressed the gas pedal and the wheels spun.

Finally, I called Steve and said, "I'm stuck in the driveway and I can't get out! I am supposed to be at my appointment in 20 minutes!" In all of his logical male wisdom, he stated I was not going to make it and needed to call and reschedule my appointment. This was not what I wanted to hear. I had been through hell the day before, setting up these appointments and dealing with insurance changes. Furthermore, I had prepped myself with the "tasty liquid" and was ready to have these tests. Putting them off would delay my treatment process another week or two. So, I did what any woman would do. I hung up on him and sat down in my driveway and cried. I needed to call someone to come and get me so I could get to the hospital for my tests, and I was running out of time.

Some friends had volunteered to take me to my appointments, but I would miss this one by the time I called them and had them pick me up. Quickly, I thought I'd try calling my neighbor. Of all days, Debbie (another angel) was off work that day! I told her what had happened and she came over and we were on our way in about five minutes. Thank God she was there! She dropped me off and I made arrangements with my mother-in-law to pick me up after I was finished with my tests.

More Insurance Drama

I approached the front desk at the hospital to register. The lady asked for my insurance information. "What is the name and policy number of your insurance?" *Gee, here comes another ordeal,* I thought. I didn't have the information but explained to her that I would have it in a few days. She asked me if I worked. "No, I don't." The registration process ended. She asked me to wait and listen for my name to be called.

Finally, my name was called. I was brought to the billing office and a lady proceeded with my "case." I explained to her that I had insurance but was waiting for my new policy and insurance card. Again, this was falling on deaf ears. I completed a waiver for my treatment that stated I was responsible for payment. After signing several such documents, I went back to the waiting room and waited for my name to be called. I felt humiliated by the assumptions the clerical staff was making during this process. I wanted to scream, "I am not trying to get a free ride! I am trying to **March Forth** to rid my breast of cancer, for God's sake! I *have* insurance! I just don't have the card with me!"

Finally, my name was called. When my tests were completed, I called my mother-in-law and she took me home. It had been an exhausting day.

Later that evening, I opened my mail. There was a

letter from my former insurance company. The letter was dated January 31, 2009—the final day of my coverage with this insurance. My BRCA1/BRCA2 tests had been denied due to a clause inserted in the policy. The letter stated I could appeal the denial. *How nice of them to offer*, I thought. I'd had no time to even begin the appeal process because the insurance had ended that day! Perfect timing on their part! Thus, the effort I'd begun on January 22, 2009, to take the BRCA1/BRCA2 tests had stalled on this date—February 4, 2009. Good gracious! I was glad when that day ended. I was exhausted and disappointed that I had been reduced to a piece of paper.

The BRCA1/BRCA2 Tests

February 5, 2009, was a new day and hopefully a new beginning after the fiasco of the day before. I received a telephone call from the lab where my BRCA1/BRCA2 tests had been sent. The lab technician told me coverage for my tests had been denied by my insurance. (Yes, I'd been informed of this yesterday!) The technician explained that if I still wanted the tests completed, they could arrange a loan to pay for them. (This loan was offered at an unbelievably high interest rate.) She had received my blood sample but had been waiting for insurance approval to process and test it. She explained that I could pay for the tests myself or complete a loan application and still have it tested. (Wow! I could see how a life-threatening illness could wipe out a person's life savings in a heartbeat. It's easy to make a bad financial decision when you're in such a fragile emotional state.)

I explained to the lab technician about our health insurance change. She advised me that if I had new insurance, most likely I would need to have another blood sample drawn. The new insurance would only recognize events on or after February 1, 2009. "Let me call my new insurance and see if it's covered," I said. "So let me get this straight. You have my blood sample from January 22, 2009, but my old insurance denied it. You need a new blood sample dated on or after February 1, 2009, for my new insurance to pay for the tests—even if it will be the same blood!?"

"Yes! That is correct," she said.

I took down the information about the loan and told her I would get back to her before the end of the day.

After calling my new insurance company, I had good news: They would cover the BRCA1/BRCA2 tests! However, in order for my new insurance to cover these tests, I would need a blood sample dated on or after February 1, 2009. The lab technician had been correct. We could not use the blood sample presently sitting in the lab!

I called my surgeon's office and requested that I have a new blood sample drawn. The receptionist requested that I come in on Monday (three days later!). I had previously wasted two weeks waiting for results to determine what I needed to do, and now I was going to have to wait three more days just for a signature and another two weeks minimum for the test results!? *Ugh!* I explained my situation and asked to speak to a nurse. She put me on hold for a few minutes.

While I was on hold, information about ways to prevent cancer streamed into my ear. "Do you know how to reduce your cancer risks?" Yes, I wanted to scream. "Did you know that no smoking (didn't smoke!), minimum alcohol (yes), exercising (did that), and eating healthy (did that, too!) reduce your risk of cancer?" Ugh! I talked back to this recording each time it asked me these inane questions. *None of those precautions had helped me!* I thought. I realized that my shock was now turning to anger.

Finally, a nurse answered the phone. I explained my situation to her. "I only need a written order from the surgeon so I can retake this blood test!" I pleaded. (Time was a factor for me. My goodness! A whole month had passed and I was starting all over again!)

My surgeon was in surgery and unavailable to sign an order. The nurse would call later that afternoon and inform me whether or not they could catch him before he left for the day. I waited for the phone call.

Finally, I received the call back from the nurse. If I could get to the lab within 30 minutes, my blood sample would make the outgoing shipment for the day. If I could not make it in time, the blood sample would need to be taken on Monday—three days later.

It was the afternoon of Friday, February 6, 2009, when I arrived at the hospital to have another blood sample drawn. The weight of this week's frustrations and anxiety was taking its toll. I lashed out mentally as a young man stood outside the hospital in the 40-degree weather with an IV attached to his arm. He was dressed only in a hospital gown and pants, smoking and holding his IV pole. I don't think this young man had any clue what he was doing to his body. *Do you want cancer too, Bud!?* He had made the <u>choice</u> to smoke. I lived a preventive life-style but I still had cancer! I was an active, healthy, ath-letic 49-year-old woman who did not smoke and rarely drank. I was in excellent health—or so I'd thought. *How did I get breast cancer!? Why isn't he helping himself!? Doesn't he know he can get cancer from smoking!? Ugh!* I went into the hospital. The lab technician took another blood sample. He personally delivered it to the shipment department, and it was sent out in time. I applaud the efforts of all the employees who helped me that day. They were my un-sung heroes, helping me to get the second blood sample sent back to the lab for the BRCA1/BRCA2 tests.

I don't understand why processing medical claims is so difficult. My veterinarian cousin summed it up best. He said, "Obviously, if your dog needed surgery, it would be completed the next day if everyone was in agreement with the procedures and cost." I couldn't help but think if I were a dog, my surgery would have been completed by now. Again, the waiting was agonizing.

While I waited, I wondered. *Was the cancer growing fast? Was it expanding?* I wanted it out of my body. I was tired of fighting through the procedures and paperwork. I called my oncologist and relayed the information about the delay on the BRCA1/BRCA2 tests. He advised me to go ahead and schedule the surgery and not wait any longer for the results.

I applaud the medical, technical, and scientific minds that created these wonderful BRCA1/BRCA2 tests to help women determine their cancer risk and treatments. These tests were created for those considered high risk for breast cancer. I'd passed the initial screening tool used to decide which patients were good candidates for them. However, it was disappointing to see the use of this wonderful technology lost in a paper shuffle. I began another wait.

On Monday, February 12, 2009, I called the surgeon's office to schedule my surgery. The surgeon was out of town and would not be available until February 19, 2009! Seven more days before any action! I was in waiting mode again. I would have wasted a whole month waiting for the results of my BRCA1/BRCA2 tests. It made me angry that my life had been reduced to paperwork during that time. No life should be reduced to a piece of paper and a few dollar bills. But, sadly enough, it happens all the time.

After I made my appointment with the surgeon, there was nothing more I could do but wait and be positive. Though I was mentally exhausted from the whole medical ordeal of the past two months, I continued to *March Forth.* When I attended social functions, well-wishers asked how I was doing. I tried to respond positively. "I'm great!" or "I am terrific!" I said. It was better than telling them I thought I was going to die. After all, I didn't have time for any negative thoughts.

On Friday, February 13, 2009, I received a phone call from the breast center. They had my BRCA1/BRCA2 results back! How could that be?! How had the information come back so quickly?! "Are you ready to hear your results?" I heard a voice ask. *Yes and no*, I thought. I closed my eyes. This was the moment I had been waiting for. I needed this information to determine my cancer treatment.

The results of my blood test drawn, on Friday, February 6, were in on February 12, 2009! Six days later! And yet I had been waiting for them for a whole month?! Had I tested positive?! Would I need the double mastectomy and oophorectomy?! My mind was cycling through all types of questions. "No mutation was detected!" the voice said. I had tested negative! I didn't have the genetic susceptibility gene for this particular type of cancer! I didn't have to have a double mastectomy or an oophorectomy! My eyes began to water and I exhaled a big sigh of relief. It was a small victory, but I still had to fight another battle. For now, I needed to get the breast with cancer removed as soon as I could. ***March Forth*** Marci, ***March Forth!***

14

FINALLY, A BETTER WEEK AHEAD

On February 19, 2009, I had two appointments: one with my surgeon and one with my oncologist. I was anxious to get to my surgeon so I could set a surgery date. I was ready to get this process moving. When the nurse entered to take my vitals, she asked if I had seen a plastic surgeon yet. "No, I have not," I said. She stated I would not be able to set up my surgery date until this was done! I was furious! Why had they not told me this before now?! She told me I would need a consultation for my reconstruction before I could have my breast removed. Whoa!" I said. "I am _not_ having reconstruction! I am having a unilateral mastectomy and that's all!" (Thankfully, that was all I was having. I would have been livid if I'd had to postpone surgery because I had not seen a plastic surgeon first. I would have wasted another 10 days waiting again. Make sure to see a plastic surgeon _before_ you schedule your final breast surgery _if_ you choose the reconstruction route.)

Finally, I met my surgeon and we discussed and finalized an action plan. He would be removing one breast and three lymph nodes during the surgery. I would be admitted to the hospital as an outpatient early in the morning on the day of my surgery for a sentinel node test. (The sentinel node surgery is less invasive and has fewer side effects than the node dissections used in the past.) I would be taken to the breast center to have a radioactive injection (sometimes a dye is used) in my breast. This injected material would gradually travel to the lymph nodes. The first lymph node it drained to would be the sentinel (first) lymph node. If the cancer had spread from the tumors in my breast, it would most likely show in the sentinel node first.

Two more lymph nodes surrounding the sentinel node would also be removed. These three lymph nodes would then be examined during my surgery. If any of the three lymph nodes tested positive for cancer cells, then more lymph nodes would be removed during the surgery for further testing. After the sentinel injection, I would be admitted to the hospital for my mastectomy. After surgery, I would be placed in a recovery room and then moved to a hospital room for observance overnight. I'd be released within 24 hours if there were no immediate problems. (I called this the Drive-by Whack-a Boob-Surgery!) After all my questions were answered, I immediately went to the receptionist to schedule my surgery date, relieved to finally have a solid action plan in front of me. I was elated to hear that my scheduled surgery date was ***Thursday, March 4, 2009!*** The final exclamation point had been placed on this journey for me.

March 4th has always been a special day for me. It is the only "action day" listed on the calendar. I love telling people March 4th is "action day." Most people look at me oddly until I explain. March 4th is "action day" because it's the only day that tells us to do something—_March Forth_. I always felt March 4th was a positive day for action. How fitting for me to have surgery on March 4th. "That date works for me!" I told the receptionist.

Following my appointment with the surgeon, I saw the oncologist. I informed him of my surgery date and my decision to have a simple unilateral mastectomy. He told me that my tests and scans were OK. My brain MRI was negative. (I already knew I had nothing left in my brain. I could have saved some money on that test!) My chest, abdominal cavity, and pelvic scans were also negative. There was a very good chance I would not need radiation since we were removing my total breast. Again, the doctor felt confident we had caught the cancer at an early stage. Further treatment would be determined from the results of the pathology report after surgery. Finally, everything was scheduled. Two more weeks and, hopefully, this ride would come to an end.

After my visit with the oncologist, I scheduled a return appointment on the Monday following my mastectomy. "We will review the pathology report and determine our course of action then," he said. He explained to me how critical the pathology report was following surgery. "The lymph nodes are a critical check during surgery," he said. "They are given a quick scan to help the surgeon decide whether more surgery is needed or more lymph nodes need to be excised. Sometimes the quick check can miss some diseased cells. That is why the pathology report is so important." The pathologist can take a section or sample of the lymph node, slice and dice it, and then scrutinize it in greater detail. "Make sure you have the results of the pathology report before assuming the lymph nodes are disease free," he said. These words rang in my ears. I would think about that statement a lot for the next two weeks.

Finally, the stage was set. All my preliminary tests had been completed. Everything was scheduled for surgery. On March 4, 2009, I would ***March Forth*** and rid my body of this dreaded disease called cancer.

15

TWO WEEKS TO PREP FOR SURGERY

For the next two weeks I rested and came to terms with what I was facing. I had not had a chance to do this yet because of the insurance hassles, paperwork, appointments, and medical tests. I kept my mind distracted and myself busy. I made plenty of phone calls.

I received many cards and prayers during this time. Our family accepted many blessings from people reaching out to us. I cannot thank all of my friends and family enough for their kindness and compassion during this crisis. Even strangers extended their hands to help us. It restored my faith in humanity.

Towards the end of February, Clay and I went to see our beloved Purdue Boilermakers play basketball at Mackey Arena. We'd received two tickets as a Christmas present. Clay and I drove to West Lafayette, Indiana for the game. Steve and Corey stayed home to help with a church function. I thought I would have to cancel this trip and knew Clay would be heartbroken if we couldn't go due to my surgery. When we'd bought the tickets in December, our family had not anticipated this disruption in our lives. So I was glad we were able to make this small getaway before my surgery.

We arrived early at Mackey Arena. Clay was approached immediately (another angel) and asked to be the Taco Bell Ball Boy for the game. Apparently, they had a no-show and Clay was in the right place at the right time. Of course, I immediately started calling everyone to tell them, "My son is the Purdue Basketball Taco Bell Ball Boy for today's game and it's being televised live by ESPN!" I went to my seat and watched proudly during the game as Clay mingled with the basketball players, cheerleaders, and Paint Crew. I saw how he beamed when he was rubbing shoulders with Purdue Pete and the camera crew. I cried. *Will I see him and Corey have other opportunities like this in the future? Will I even see them graduate from high school? Will I see them graduate from college, possibly Purdue University, where Clay says he wants to study? Will I see them grow up to be men?* Clay was smiling—something he had rarely done the last two months. He was having a transitional year in grade school and it was being complicated by my situation. He was very much worried about me, but now he was enjoying himself immensely. These Purdue students (more angels) were touching my son's life and had no clue how important they were at this point in time. It was a much-needed mental boost for both of us. His excitement was still bubbling over as we left for home after the game. He chirped about all the encounters he'd had during the ball game. Before we were 30 minutes outside of West Lafayette, he was sound asleep. I drove home alone with my thoughts. It was a memorable moment for both of us, with hopefully a lot more to come. ***March Forth***, Clay, ***March Forth!***

16

MARCH (FORTH) 4TH: SURGERY DAY

Finally, March 4, 2009, arrived. I awoke early to take my son Corey to the orthodontist. This would help distract me from the events that lay ahead that day.

Corey was my internal child. I wasn't sure how he was coping with the events of the last two months because he was a young man of few words. He is my firstborn.

Fourteen years earlier, I was having trouble becoming pregnant and had finally accepted the fact that I was unable to have children. Thus, I changed jobs at work and took a supervisor's position. I had been working long hours on a start-up project and thought that was why I was so tired. Still, just in case, I bought an over-the-counter pregnancy test. I took the test, and as I watched the indicator change color, my immediate thought was not that I was going to have a baby but *I'm going to have a boy!* (I'm not sure how I knew.) I was thrilled I was going to be a mom!

I carried Corey through one of the hottest summers on record. I dealt with the heat and gestational high blood pressure all summer long. Late summer, Steve and I moved to a new home. During the middle of our move, my water broke. Corey arrived 3½ weeks early but healthy. He also **_Marched Forth_** and thrived after his birth.

❧❧

With the orthodontist appointment concluded, I took Corey to school and came home. I collected my personal items and Steve and I left for the hospital. An hour later, I was admitted as an outpatient. Finally, after two months, I was "fixing" the problem.

I was nervous, concerned about the length of the surgery, concerned about the anesthesia, and I was sad that I was going to lose my breast. However, as traumatic as these things were for me, I was most concerned about my lymph nodes. It was critical for me not to have any diseased lymph nodes.

My mother had had several lymph nodes removed during her mastectomy. As a result, she'd had a few bouts with lymphedema. She'd also had cellulitis a couple of times because her lymph system was compromised. Each time she had cellulitis, she ended up in the hospital fighting this serious infection of the tissues. I did not want this to happen to me. And I did not want any more than the three scheduled lymph nodes removed. Furthermore, if more diseased lymph nodes were found, it meant I had a more advanced stage of cancer than we'd originally thought.

I registered at the hospital and gave them my living will. (Yes! I have an insurance card!) I was wheeled back to a holding room and prepped for my sentinel node test.

While waiting for the transporter, I was concerned about my father showing up for my surgery. He would have to walk a great distance to get to the holding room where I was stationed. Dad felt he needed to be there for me. He was 82 years old and had experienced more than his fair share of medical challenges, fighting back each time. He never gave up and continued to do the best he could. Walking was sometimes a challenge for him due to a previous stroke, but he always managed to get where he needed to be. However, he had still not arrived at that point.

A transporter came and I was wheeled to the breast center for my sentinel node test. I had the same technician that I had during my biopsy. I was glad she was there. She had been informative and caring throughout my previous biopsy procedure.

The radioactive material was injected under the nipple and near the tumor. (This injection was slightly painful.) It was now up to the radioactive material to travel to a lymph node for filtering. The first lymph node that the radioactive material went to would be the sentinel node, which the surgeon would find with a Geiger counter.

I was transported back to the hospital to my holding room. Steve was waiting for me. I was then admitted into the hospital. My minister arrived shortly after my return. I was concerned Dad would miss me before I was wheeled away for surgery. Finally, he showed up with my aunt and uncle (Dad's brother). My aunt had brought them to the hospital. They all were exhausted from walking the long distance to where I was located. I was glad they finally made it because I was worried about Dad getting too exhausted.

The small holding room was starting to overflow with people. Within a few minutes after Dad arrived, the transporter wheeled me off for my 2:00 p.m. surgery. I said my prayers as I was wheeled away. I was scared about the surgery, about losing my breast, and about the possibility of finding more diseased lymph nodes. However, the "party" started as I felt the anesthesia begin to take hold. ***March Forth***, Marci, ***March Forth!***

The first thing I recall after being wheeled into the recovery room was one nurse communicating to another. I heard "left mastectomy lymph nodes negative." *Was she talking about me?* I was starting to get my bearings, but my eyes would not open. I didn't want to wake up because I was in such a restful state. The medical staff were moving and talking around me. I remember the feeling of warm blankets being placed upon me. They were comforting. I felt like my body was trying to turn to the right side as I lay on the bed. It made me dizzy, and I felt a little disoriented. Finally, I thought maybe it was my body trying to rebalance itself since my breast was gone. I felt for my breast. It _was_ gone. Finally, I was conscious enough to ask, "Did they take more lymph nodes?" "No," the nurse said. "The lymph nodes were negative." What a relief! My eyes watered. That was good news! That meant no more diseased lymph nodes! We did catch the cancer early! *I am now cancer free,* I thought! *I can move forward.* I had no regrets now about losing my breast. I had to remove it in order to save my life.

My pain was manageable as they wheeled me to my hospital room. I was still under the anesthesia, but it was wearing off. Steve, Dad, Uncle Art, and Aunt Rose were waiting for me. I didn't feel like talking much, but they wanted to see me and make sure I was situated before they went home. I remember being keenly aware of an odor. Some type of cleaning chemical was making me nauseous. I wanted to sleep.

Three hours later, I was able to talk to visitors. I had been kidding all week about having a margarita to help me get through the surgery. My friend Doris visited me later that evening and brought me a get well card from her and my friend Sandy. It held a gift card to the local Mexican restaurant that serves the best margaritas in town. I started laughing. Doris did not know why. How fitting that she brought me that gift card! I explained how she and Sandy (more angels) had sent just the right gift at the right time.

My wonderful friend Carolyn, who had helped so much in the last two months, brought Corey and Clay to the hospital. I wanted my sons to see me after surgery so they'd know I was OK. After a short visit, I sent the boys and Steve home. I knew Steve was very tired. It had been a long day for everyone. (Sometimes I think managing a health crisis is harder on the caregiver than the care receiver.) After they went home, I slept.

Around 11:00 p.m., the pain in my arm grew

significantly. The mastectomy site was not too painful but, my upper arm where the lymph nodes had been removed hurt badly. It felt like I had a rope tied around my upper arm and someone was tightening it. I paged the nurse and asked for my pain medication. I wanted to make sure I stayed medicated ahead of the pain.

I awoke around 2:00 a.m., restless. I unplugged my IV machine and started walking around the hallway. I wanted to build my strength up as quickly as I could. Two laps around the nurses' station exhausted me. I crawled back into the hospital bed and slept until early morning.

Early the next morning, I was awakened by the nurses. They gave me my pain medication, checked my vitals, and drained the bulb that was connected to a tube inserted in the surgical site on my chest. The bulb was squeezed, then capped, to create a slight suction in the tube. The suction pulled the accumulating fluid around the surgical site into the bulb. Surgeons usually attach one or two bulbs per breast removed. I had one bulb inserted in my surgical area.

Midmorning my surgeon arrived and examined my surgical site. He stated I was healing nicely and that my cancer diagnosis was considered stage I because no lymph nodes were involved. (Stage I had a 95 percent survival rate for five years.) He showed me how to empty my bulb and then released me from the hospital. I called Steve and told him to come and pick me up. I showered and dressed myself, then waited for Steve. I was released from the hospital around 11:30 a.m. Home was waiting for me. ***March Forth, Marci!***

17

THE PATHOLOGY REPORT

On Monday, March 9, 2009, four days after my surgery, I went to my oncologist appointment. I was still feeling puny from my surgery. Steve drove me to the doctor's office. The oncologist was going to review my pathology report and discuss treatment options based on the report. I couldn't help but recall what he'd said about the lymph nodes at my last visit. My final hurdle was standing in front of me: My pathology report would be the final verdict as to on whether or not my lymph nodes were diseased with cancer.

When we entered the office, I watched and waited as the doctor settled into his chair. He began reviewing the pathology report.

"The pathologist found one small tumor in one of the three lymph nodes," he said. Both Steve and I sank in our chairs. The oncologist stated that it was not uncommon to find a tumor in the lymph nodes after surgery because the pathologist is able to scrutinize the sample in greater detail. He said it was not unusual for lobular cancer to "jump around" like mine had to the lymph node. *I was now looking at full-blown chemotherapy treatment for 20 weeks!*

How could this be when the tumors were so small? How could I be so sick that I needed 20 weeks of chemotherapy? I still felt healthy, although I had been very tired the last few months leading up to my diagnosis. This process was taking a mental toll. The doctor told me I was going to lose my hair. That was the least of my worries. Questions and thoughts began tumbling through my mind. Had the cancer traveled somewhere else and the technology not found it? I stopped my thoughts and tried to listen. I needed to meet with the chemotherapy nurse before I started my treatments. She would review what I needed to do and how to take care of myself during the chemotherapy.

"Do I need to go back for more surgery to remove more lymph nodes as a result of the pathology report?" I asked. My oncologist said it would not be necessary for two reasons: The tumor found in the lymph node was very small and encased. It was in its beginning stage. Second, the status of my lymph nodes determined the course of my treatment. The 20 weeks of chemotherapy was the most treatment I could endure at this point. My outlook was still good, but I was now considered to have Stage II cancer, with an 85 percent survival rate for five years. My odds of survival decreased 10 percent during this doctor's appointment!

We left the doctor's office and made an appointment with the chemotherapy nurse. I was discouraged. I became angry on the way home. *If we hadn't wasted so much time on the insurance,* I thought, *maybe this would not have happened.* But I did not want to look backwards. I wanted to look forwards. I needed to _**March Forth!**_

I was extremely glad I had made the decision to remove the whole breast, especially after reading the pathology report. The pathologist had found lobular cancer in situ (LCIS). These cells were classified as precancerous cells that had a high likelihood of turning into lobular cancer cells, and they had not appeared on my scans.

I went home and took another pain pill. I had been knocked down again. I had to get my breath back and get my "legs" underneath me. I was not feeling well because of the surgery. It had only been four days! It was hard to swallow what I'd heard today. However, I had to battle on and I needed to gather some strength so I could _**March Forth.**_

18

IN LIMBO, WAITING FOR CHEMO

After my surgery, several friends and family members wanted to help me and my family in some way. Many wanted to bring food. Several called and asked what they could do for me. I was overwhelmed by what had transpired over the last few weeks, and the big lymph node bombshell had scattered my senses. I couldn't concentrate. The smallest task was overpowering me. However, I quickly saw that I needed to organize a meal schedule in some way to help my family, especially now that I was going to have chemotherapy.

Steve and I enjoyed helping others. However, sometimes our pride prevented us from letting others help us in return. We were not comfortable with accepting and receiving help. But I was finally learning that if people want to help, let them! Helping prevents your friends from feeling helpless. It also can soothe the anger of helplessness. It can provide a much-needed service for you and your family when your world has been rocked. Our friends and family wanted to help. No one could take the pain or cancer away, but I realize we needed to let others help us.

Thus, I asked my friend Valerie to help organize a meal schedule. I sent an e-mail to our friends and family explaining that Valerie was organizing this task for our family. We requested that she schedule meals every other day and not on weekends. Those who wanted to help responded to her. She set up a schedule with names and phone numbers in case there was a conflict. She then gave us the schedule. This task was so appreciated, and the response of our friends and family was overwhelming. We were extremely thankful for all of the caring cards, food, and prayers we received during our time of need.

On March 12, 2009, I returned to my surgeon for my follow-up visit. He removed the bulb and draining tube from the mastectomy site and removed half of the staples (approximately 10) from my incision site. I thought the metal table would melt from the hot grip of my hands as he plucked the staples from my incision. That was painful, to say the least. Each one was worse as I anticipated the pull from the tool he was using. I was caught off guard when he began and did not recover until he was finished. I had been trying to wean myself off the pain medicine, and if I had known it was going to be that painful, I would have taken one of my pain pills before I went in. Anyway, he said I was healing nicely.

We discussed the pathology report. I relayed the information I had received from my oncologist. Removing more lymph nodes was discussed but not recommended due to the full chemotherapy treatment I was going to receive. I was scheduled to return to the surgeon the following week to have the remaining staples in my chest removed.

That day, following the surgeon's visit, I had my consultation with the chemotherapy nurse. She gave me information about each drug and described its purpose and effects. I would be taking Adriamycin, Cytoxan, and Taxol. It was called the ACT treatment. I would receive four combined treatments of the Adriamycin and Cytoxan. These two drugs would stop the growth of cancer cells and this drug combination would be given every two weeks. Called the "Red Devil Cocktail", it had some major side effects: decreased white blood cell count, decreased platelets, loss of appetite, darkening of nail beds, hair loss, nausea, vomiting, and blood in the urine, acne, tiredness, and sores in the mouth or on the lips. Some severe side effects included changes in electrocardiogram (EKG), irregular heartbeat, heart damage with congestive heart failure, and scarring of lung tissue, causing a cough and shortness of breath. Whew! And these were only the side effects listed!

After the four treatments of Adriamycin and Cytoxan, I would receive 12 treatments of Taxol once a week. This drug stops cell division, resulting in cell death. The major side effects of Cytoxan were decreased white blood cell count with increased risk of infection, tiredness and fatigue, numbness and tingling in hands and/or feet, irritation of nerves, muscle and bone aches, hair loss, nausea, vomiting, mild diarrhea, and mild stomatitis (inflammation of the mucous tissue lining the mouth). This drug had an increased chance of an allergic reaction (rarely) causing anaphylaxis. In addition to these side effects, I had other precautions and activities I would need to avoid or watch.

The nurse explained I that would also need to do the following:

- I needed a portacath or port catheter (port) inserted in my clavicle area for administering my chemotherapy. The nurse would contact my surgeon and schedule the outpatient surgery. This port needed to be inserted before I started my chemotherapy treatments.
- During treatments, I needed to drink plenty of fluids each day. The chemotherapy drugs dry out your body. Therefore, I needed to drink a minimum of 80 ounces a day! (I set a goal to drink 100 ounces a day.)
- If at any time I had a small fever, I needed to immediately contact the nurse. The chemotherapy would drop my white blood cell count; therefore, it was imperative that I contact the doctor immediately if I got a cold or got sick.
- She advised me to take extra vitamin B6 to help with anemia and neuropathy. Furthermore, she checked the vitamins and supplements I was presently taking to make sure they did not conflict with the chemotherapy. (It's important to do this because some vitamins and supplements can interfere with the chemotherapy.)
- I needed to keep food in my stomach to help reduce

nausea and maintain my weight.
- Light exercise would also be beneficial.

The information was overwhelming. My brain was overloaded as I sat and listened to the informative but straightforward nurse. This chemo stuff was serious and scary.

As I was listening, my thoughts raced. I couldn't believe I was taking chemotherapy treatments. My memory flashed back to my mom and her treatments. It had absolutely killed me the first time I saw the needle go into her arm, especially when the chemicals drained into her body. I thought about how the chemo drugs were going to destroy her. Now, they were going to destroy me. However, I had chosen this solution. So I listened and decided to heed the nurse and doctor's advice. Mom was brave and I can be brave, too. Our consultation ended and I went home.

On March 16, 2009, I went to the heart hospital to have an echocardiogram (EKG) to test my heart function, since the Adriamycin in large quantities can injure the heart muscle. My EKG was normal; therefore, I had the green light to receive the Adriamycin. Later in the day, the oncology nurse called to inform me that my port surgery was scheduled for March 18, 2009—two days away. My first surgeon was out of town again; therefore, a new surgeon would place the port in my chest. We had less than a week before my chemotherapy began, and it would be beneficial for me to have the port implanted beforehand.

I still needed to purchase a wig and find my prosthesis.

I hadn't felt well enough to go out and shop and was not really sure where to find these items. During my oncology nurse consultation, I found information on a wig shop. I made plans the next day to go with a friend to get my wig. It was my last free day before my port surgery and I knew I wouldn't feel well after it because I still hadn't fully recovered from the mastectomy.

The next day my friend Carolyn and I went to buy my wig. We had some fun as I tried on different colors and styles, laughing at some of my possible new looks. I selected a wig that I thought was totally me. However, the stylist selected a wig for me as well. I tried mine on first. It was awful! I then tried the stylist's selection. It was perfect.

It's important to purchase a wig before you lose your hair. The stylist is a professional and can closely match your natural hair, but she needs to see your present hairstyle to help select a wig that is right for you. Lesson learned.

After I selected my wig, I chose one head cover from several selections. (My insurance did not cover hair loss; therefore I purchased conservatively.) A person could easily overspend in one of these shops. It is an emotional journey to lose your hair during treatments. But, buying several head covers would not prevent my hair loss. I decided I could come back after experiencing my hair loss to purchase more items if needed.

Many organizations donate free head covers and wigs to cancer patients who lose their hair. A lady from my church who belongs to the local sewing guild gave me a head cover. The guild makes and donates head covers for local cancer patients. You can find these services through your local oncology office or American Cancer Society.

While I was at the wig shop, I mentioned that I still needed my prosthesis but didn't know where to find a specialty shop. The stylist told me where I could find these specialty items. Carolyn and I went there immediately and scheduled my fitting for the morning before my first chemotherapy treatment.

Later, I went home and checked with my insurance company to make sure the specialty shop was "in network." Wouldn't you know it; the specialty shop was "out of network." I contacted the insurance nurse assigned to my case. She obtained an exception so that the specialty shop qualified as "in network" for my insurance. My insurance carrier didn't carry any local specialty shops that were "in network."

The next day (March 19, 2009), I went to the hospital for my outpatient port surgery. I had not met my surgeon yet, which was causing me anxiety. We had to squeeze this outpatient surgery into my schedule so my port would be inserted before my first chemotherapy treatment and this was the only time that would fit into the surgeon's and my schedule.

I had to find information about my new surgeon, but it was limited. She had recently moved into the area to begin her practice. While I was being prepped for my outpatient surgery, she finally arrived and introduced herself. We reviewed the details of my surgery: I would be placed under anesthesia for the insertion of my port or tube in a large vein just off center from my collarbone. The port would remain in my chest until the chemotherapy treatments were completed or until the oncologist released the port for removal. (Some ports remain in the chest several years; my port would remain for several months.

The chemotherapy drugs are administered through the head or port of the tube. The port is inserted and lies just under the skin. It appears as a small bump under the skin about the size of a quarter on the chest wall. The nurses can easily access the port and insert IVs to administer chemotherapy drugs and there is less discomfort to the patient from administering chemotherapy via the port. The port would also serve as an easy access point for the bloodwork I needed before each chemotherapy treatment. (Some doctors do not allow this.) If a patient is scheduled for several chemotherapy treatments, a port is highly recommended.

After the port was inserted, the surgeon would remove the remaining staples in my chest from the mastectomy surgery. (What a relief that I would not have to be awake to experience that tender pain of having those staples removed again!) I instantly liked the surgeon and felt confident that my surgery would be successful. This was a good feeling before going under the anesthesia.

Finally, the transporter arrived and carted me to the operating room for surgery. Again, I faced the cold surgery room with the big white light. I was asked to count backwards from 10 to one. The next thing, I was waking up in the recovery room with my port inserted and my remaining staples removed. I was scheduled for a follow-up appointment and sent home. Another surgery completed.

I returned to the surgeon's office two days later so she could examine the area of my port. I still was not feeling well from my mastectomy two weeks earlier. My arm was hurting down to my wrist, where it felt like a tendon had been wound very tightly. I couldn't flex my wrist backwards, and my nerves were irritated, which made me agitated. I was still trying to wean myself off the pain medication. (I wanted to be free of it by the time I started chemotherapy treatments.)

When I entered the examination room, a nurse came forward to take my vitals. She also wanted to take my blood pressure. (After a mastectomy, vitals must be taken in the arm opposite the mastectomy. If lymph nodes have been removed, the bloodflow can be compromised in the arm closest to the site. All blood pressure readings and needle sticks need to be taken in the opposite arm or even an ankle in the case of a double mastectomy.) As the nurse approached me to take my vitals, she asked, "Which arm is your cancer arm?" I looked at her, completely offended. I was taken aback by her audacity and insensitivity. I replied, "I do not have a cancer arm! I do not have cancer. The cancer was removed from my body when I had my mastectomy and lymph node dissection! My mastectomy was on the left side of my body, if that is what you want to know." I told her I considered myself cancer free at this point. (*How dare she insinuate that I had cancer?!* I thought.)

I don't think she realized how offensive her bedside manner was to me. Nor do I think she intended it to be. However, she is a professional and surely she needed to review her sensitivity training. Hopefully, she learned from that encounter so another patient would not face those insensitive remarks. (***March Forth***, sister!!)

After my port surgery follow-up, I went home. I was hurting. My arm hurt from the mastectomy. The nerves in my arm were irritated. The surgical wound from my port insertion was throbbing. And I was having an anesthesia hangover.

I wanted to lie down. But I couldn't lie on my back because my low back was hurting. If I lay down on my left side, my mastectomy site hurt. If I lay on my right side the skin near the port on my chest pulled. I definitely could not lie on my stomach because of the mastectomy and port. I was stuck. I wanted to rest, but how?

I went to sit on my big comfy couch and took another pain pill. After a small rest, I gathered some strength and went to soak in the bathtub. I lay in the bathtub with my agony and prepared myself for Monday, March 23, 2009. In two more days, I would begin my chemotherapy treatments. I felt terrible. *How am I going to get through this when I feel so bad right now? How am I going to heal when the chemotherapy is going to kill my healthy cells?* For now, I was going to soak in the bathtub. For now, I only had to concentrate on the present. For now, I was clear of cancer. My diseased breast and lymph node had been removed. My scans and tests proved this! *Don't let your mind wander from that thought,* I told myself. Two days to rest—not in my bed, perhaps, but sitting on my comfy couch. I needed this rest before I **_Marched Forth_** to the next battle that was waiting for me Monday—my first chemotherapy treatment.

19

CHEMOTHERAPY—
THE INTERNAL/EXTERNAL CLIMB

My First "Red Devil Cocktail" Treatment

On Monday, March 23, 2009, I went to my prosthesis fitting and walked out with a new breast. I was elated. I could not believe how it molded to my body. It became a part of me as if I had never lost my breast. The texture was almost the same as my real breast. (Technology had evolved significantly since my mother's era!) I could not be more pleased with it. It also was a big boost for my mental state.

It had been two and a half weeks since my mastectomy, and I was beginning to feel better physically. However, I needed a breast. I was starting to become self-conscious about the missing breast, but now the prosthesis made me feel whole again. It helped my mood tremendously.

Although my mastectomy site was tender, I was able to wear the prosthesis. It was at this point that I realized I still had some sensation at the mastectomy site. Apparently, this was why I had hurt so badly when the surgeon removed my staples. Most women are numb in this area after a mastectomy, even more so and especially after reconstruction surgery. Thus, I was extremely grateful I had not chosen reconstruction, especially now that I was facing chemotherapy treatments.

After my prosthesis fitting, I came home to prepare for my chemotherapy treatment. I packed a jacket, a prayer shawl given to me by a local church, and earphones for my music. I would use these items during the four-hour chemotherapy infusion treatment. I also packed my two prescriptions for nausea. I would later learn I needed to apply a prescription cream to the port area to numb it. This numbing cream would deaden the sharp, painful prick when the nurse inserted the needle to administer the chemo.

The nausea medicine was a fairly new treatment for chemotherapy. I was scheduled to take two pills daily for three days beginning after my chemotherapy treatment. Some chemotherapy drugs cause more nausea than others. I had been forewarned that the Adriamycin and Cytoxan could create nausea.

Each time I would arrive for a chemotherapy treatment, I would have a blood sample taken and tested before seeing the oncologist. The blood test or CBC (complete blood count) results would determine whether I was healthy enough to have the chemotherapy that day. I was advised to wait until my test results were approved before taking the antinausea medicines. If I didn't pass the lab test, I couldn't have chemotherapy and therefore wouldn't need these expensive medicines.

I ate a light lunch and waited for Steve to come home from work. He was my rock. He had scheduled vacation time from work to be at every chemotherapy treatment and oncology appointment. I was very thankful that he was able to be with me and wanted to be there for me. He is the love of my life and a great supporter. Soon he came home and we left for my first treatment.

When I arrived for my appointment, the ritual began: sign in; pay the co-pay; and ask for copies of my lab results, scans, or tests; wait for my name to be called; weigh in; take vitals; take the CBC test; and see the doctor. If my CBC results passed, I would proceed to the infusion area, where they would administer the chemotherapy. Each week when I went to my appointment, the receptionist would ask me how I was doing and each week I would respond "terrific!" whether I felt like it or not. Then, I saw the doctor and proceeded into the infusion room to receive my chemotherapy treatment.

I sat in one of the many lounging chairs to receive my first chemotherapy treatment. I saw one of the nurses who had treated my mom! It was an emotional day for me.

For the past three months I had been poked, prodded, cut, and squashed. I was beginning to develop a fear of needles. In the past, whenever I was getting pricked in my arm, I could turn my head and look the other way. But now, I suddenly realized that the needlestick was going to happen right in front of my face, under my chin! I panicked and thought about grabbing the nurse's hands before she inserted the needle. She realized I was anxious and asked me to take a deep breath. From that day on, when I was preparing for an infusion, I would ask the nurse to tell me when to take a deep breath before inserting the needle.

For now, it was time to access my port. The nurse cleaned the area and inserted a needle that felt as big as a pencil! I thought I was going to jump out of my chair. I broke out in a cold sweat. The port area was still tender from surgery and the needlestick hurt like crazy. It was at this point the nurse asked me if I had applied my numbing cream. I didn't understand. She explained that I could apply prescription Lidocaine cream to the port area, to make the skin numb when the port was going to be accessed. I would need to apply it approximately 45 minutes before hand. I had a prescription for the cream before I left the infusion room that day!

I chose Monday afternoons to have my chemotherapy. This allowed Steve to go to work in the morning and clear up items that had surfaced over the weekend. (Sometimes he would have to go back to work after my treatments.) By having the treatments on Mondays, I hoped to feel better by the following weekends.

It took approximately four to five hours to see the oncologist and infuse the chemotherapy drugs into my body for each treatment. For future visits, I would arrive 30 to 45 minutes earlier than my scheduled appointment so I could have my port accessed. The nurses would prep my port for chemotherapy and also grab a blood sample for analysis. This process allowed me only one needlestick per visit and shortened the prep time and wait for my infusion.

The nurse attached the IV to my port. First I would receive fluids, some more antinausea medicines, and then the Red Devil Cocktail, which is a combination of Adriamycin and Cytoxan. The Adriamycin had a reddish tint; thus the name "Red Devil Cocktail." As I mentioned earlier, Adriamycin in large quantities can damage the heart and Cytoxan can cause bleeding in the bladder. The chemicals also dehydrate the body's cells. That's why it's important to receive IV fluids during chemotherapy and drink plenty of fluids during and after.

As the fluids and drugs dripped into my body, I was scared and anxious. I took the two prescribed antinausea pills. I focused on drinking fluids to keep my bladder flushed. I wondered how I would know if I have blood in my urine since the Adriamycin's reddish tint might turn my urine red. Hmmm! I was very concerned about the quantities of the drugs I would receive. I had always been very sensitive to drugs, usually taking half the dose listed on the medication label. Yet here I was receiving the standard chemotherapy treatment for *my* diagnosis. I was traveling into the unknown.

After four hours of treatment, it was time to go home. I had one Red Devil Cocktail down and three to go. I was scheduled to return in 24 hours to have a booster shot to increase my production of white blood cells which would help prevent infections. Steve and I walked to the car and went home.

When I came home, I immediately filled up a large glass of ice water and sat on my comfy couch. I forced myself to drink fluids. I did not want to get behind on my fluids even though I already felt waterlogged from the IV fluids. I didn't want to do much but sit. I was expecting a more immediate disabling effect from the chemo, but I soon found the process was a slow burn and churn. I was starting to get a headache, which became worse as the night wore on. Several hours later, my head was hurting badly from my forehead to my temples, with no relief in sight.

As the night progressed, my stomach began to burn and it felt like I was going to have diarrhea. I catnapped on the couch throughout the night while trying to push the fluids. Even though I did not want to drink, I tried to drink as much as I could. My mouth was extremely dry. The night's darkness began to lighten. Morning was approaching.

Midmorning the next day, I started feeling very nauseated. I immediately took the two prescribed antinausea medications. I was tired and had no appetite. My headache had not lifted and I continued to feel as if something was squeezing my brain. My vision was blurry. I couldn't read because my eyes would not focus. My head continued to hurt. I watched television for the most part, drank fluids, and catnapped. Later that afternoon, my friend Erum drove me to the doctor's office for the shot that would boost my white blood cell count. I returned home and began to feel worse. It felt as if someone had a branding iron pressed against the insides of my body. I thought of a song popular back when I was in high school—"Disco Inferno," with its "Burn Baby Burn", chorus. Any humor would have helped at that point.

Forty-eight hours after my chemotherapy treatment, my body entered a torturous session of headache, nausea, and burning. It was pure hell! I began shaking. The chemotherapy was affecting my nervous system. I became light-headed and dizzy in addition to feeling the burning sensation in my stomach. I went to the bathroom to rinse my mouth out with peroxide and salt water. My mouth was developing a sore and I needed to make sure I kept it from getting infected. The nurse was very adamant about mouth hygiene.

I looked in the mirror. I was pitiful. I started brushing my hair because I knew I was going to lose it soon. My doctor told me I would lose it after my first treatment. As I was brushing my hair (I don't know how I did this, but I did), I accidently poked my eye with the prong of the brush. It brought me to my knees. It felt as if the prong were stuck in my eye. I couldn't open my eye or move it without excruciating pain. I waited 10 minutes before I could open my eye. My vision was blurry from the chemo but I was glad my eye didn't contain a prong. (It was lying in the sink.) I called my eye doctor, explained my condition and requested an antibiotic to prevent an infection. He told me the eyes have little tolerance for pain but heal quickly. He called a prescription in to the pharmacy and Steve picked it up for me on his way home from work. I went back to my comfy couch and sat. All I could do was sit, keep my eyes closed, and concentrate on the good things in my life.

I comforted myself by talking and praying to God. I

asked Him for strength and healing. As miserable as I was feeling, I knew there were a lot of other people in the world who were suffering more than I. This was going to be short term, I told myself. My chances of survival at this point were very good. I had my children, my husband, and a home. I just had to get through this second, then the next second, and so on. Steve came home from work later and helped me apply the eye medicine. Later in the evening, my eye felt better.

Chemotherapy takes you to hell's door. It's a very rough ride on a path that slides and spirals downward, beating you down physically and mentally after each treatment. The ride allows you to escape the punishment and heal briefly in time to return for another treatment. It strips you mentally and physically to the very core of your soul and what feels like the very last second of your life. Once you have entered that second, it becomes very expansive. NOTHING else matters! You really don't know where you are going or care where you have been. You could care less if you were buck naked before the world. You just want to make it through that second so you can face the next.

It was at this point I walked and talked with God. I felt His presence helping me through a second here and there, during the times I could no longer help myself. We patched the pieces of time together to form a bridge to the next second. It was a great triumph to get by each second of this nauseous state and physical pain. Praise God for He was with me! He gave me the strength to cross the bridge to the next second when I felt I was slipping.

He never let go of me. When I look back at this point in my treatment, I can see where He carried me more than I thought. It was awesome, feeling His power. It was a very humbling experience. God was my "bridge over troubled water" when pain was all around me. God and I *Marched Forth* together!

20

FIRST CHEMOTHERAPY TREATMENT RECOVERY

Each time I took the Red Devil Cocktail, I divided the two weeks following the treatment into two sessions. The first week/session was the drug and pain week and the second week/session was the recovery week. My drug and pain week was basically a week of burning, pain, nausea, and exhaustion. The recovery week was an attempt to physically achieve something: laundry, chores, bills, and maybe a short walk.

I soon found the smallest tasks were exhausting. One of these tasks was the laundry. The laundry room was in the basement. Climbing and descending the stairs exhausted me. Thus, we handed the chore over to our eldest son, Corey.

Although there were a few bumps in the learning process, he did a great job. One of his more challenging laundry tasks was hanging the shirts on the hangers correctly. Sometimes he would hang the shirts inside-out. Sometimes he didn't get the buttons in the right holes. And sometimes he didn't put the hangers through the sleeves correctly. The latter caused one of the most humorous incidents during my treatment. After explaining many times how to hang a shirt, we saw it finally hit home one day. Corey had washed one of my shirts and put it on a hanger, again missing the sleeves. By the time it dried, the hanger had created a protrusion on the left side of my shirt where my breast used to be. I put the shirt on and went to show Corey. Steve, Corey, and Clay were in the same room when I arrived. I asked if anyone noticed anything wrong with my shirt. They looked at me and snickered. Then we all had a good laugh. Needless to say, I think he finally got it. Actions sometimes do speak louder than words.

On the sixth day (Saturday) following my Red Devil Cocktail treatment, my body began to have some reprieve from the *constant* burning and nausea. However, my headache and blurry vision continued. One minute I felt better, and then the next minute I felt worse. I was recovering.

The pain and burning continued at different degrees and stages each consecutive day. The pain and nausea would ease in intensity but never go away completely. I would later learn that the pain and nausea never go away until you complete your chemotherapy treatments. For the first time since my initial treatment, I moved from my comfy couch to my bed to sleep. I finally could rest in small increments through the night.

On the seventh day following my Red Devil Cocktail treatment (Sunday night), I began to feel worse. It felt as if my heart was pumping out of my chest. I felt more light-headed and out of sync than I had all week. I called my oncologist's after-hours emergency number and explained my symptoms. They told me if I thought I was having a heart attack I needed to get to the emergency room at the hospital. I did not feel as if I was having a heart attack, so I dismissed the idea of going to the emergency room. I didn't have the energy to go anyway. Besides, my family was already in bed. I stayed up and tried to relax. I thought maybe I was having an anxiety attack.

Finally, I took my blood pressure and found it was extremely low. It was dropping below 90/60. I now deduced that maybe my heart was beating faster to try to raise my blood pressure. I stayed awake that night, afraid to go to sleep. I kept tabs on my blood pressure all night. I told myself if I felt worse, I would get Steve out of bed and go to the hospital. I was afraid I was going to pass out.

Finally, on the eighth day posttreatment (Monday morning), I called the oncology nurse. She told me to get into the office immediately, that I was dehydrated and needed fluids. *Dehydrated!* I thought. *How could I be dehydrated?!* I had been drinking anywhere from 100 to 120 ounces per day all week! (I kept a daily tally of my fluid intake on my organization board.)

I called my friend Brenda and asked her to take me to the doctor's office. When we arrived, we went to the infusion room. The nurse inserted the fluids by IV into my port. The fluids built the pressure back up in my veins and in turn raised my blood pressure. After a couple of hours of fluids, Brenda brought me home. I did feel better. However, I was aghast at what this chemotherapy could do to my body.

That evening, I felt like eating something. It was the first time I'd had an appetite. I was grateful some friends had brought us food. I was weak, and cooking was a giant task for me. Besides, the smell of food cooking made me nauseous.

I continued to recover on days 8-12 following my first chemotherapy treatment. I was getting stronger feeling better for longer time periods. On day 12, I felt well enough to drive short distances. The blurriness in my eyes had cleared enough for me to drive. However, the exhaustion was so overpowering that one small trip would wipe me out completely for the day. I would have to sleep or rest most of the day if I needed to make a trip. If I needed an appointment, I had to plan it on the 12th to 14th day following my treatment.

On the 14th day following my treatment (Sunday evening), I was beginning to feel a lot better. However, it was a big reality check. The very next day would be my second Red Devil Cocktail. My mental state began to plummet because I was now faced with repeating the two-week nightmare. My anxiety was starting to build at the thought of it. *How was I going to get through another treatment?* I thought. *The first two weeks of this treatment had been hell!* I could not imagine going through another two weeks like I'd just gone through. But I had to do it. I had three more of these "Devils". I would have to find the strength because treatment number two was staring me in the face in 24 hours. (I was going to face the same side effects I went through the previous two weeks!) Again, I reminded myself that I just needed to focus on the present. It was all I had to accomplish. *Focus on now,* I thought.

I went to shower. My head had been tingling the last few days. I had been losing several strands of hair all week. But now, as I ran my fingers through my hair, large clumps of it rested in the palm of my hand. The time had arrived. I was going to lose my hair. I needed to wash my hair but I knew if I did, it was going to fall out and fill my bathtub. I decided to leave my hair alone. I would not shampoo or brush my hair until tomorrow evening, after my second treatment.

I went back to my comfy couch. I needed to concentrate on the now—not tomorrow. I needed to focus on how much better I felt now than a few days ago. I had a few hours of good before the bad would begin again. I searched for something positive and tried to keep the negative thoughts out of my head. I had to rest and enjoy NOW because I was in less pain. I had to focus on the present moment, not tomorrow's sting. *__March forth__* for now, Marci. *__March Forth!__*

21

HAIR TODAY, GONE TOMORROW!

My Second "Red Devil Cocktail" Treatment

The next morning was Monday, April 6, 2009. Two weeks had passed since my first treatment. I began my ritual of preparation for my second Red Devil Cocktail. I packed my jacket, prayer shawl, earphones, and nausea medicines and applied the numbing cream to my port area. I ate brunch an egg sandwich and milk. (I wanted orange juice but due to the acid in the juice, I couldn't drink it. The acid hurt my stomach.)

I put a scarf on my head and wrapped it tightly around my hair. I waited for Steve to come home from work and take me to the doctor's office. When we arrived at the doctor's office, the ladies greeted me at the front desk. They asked me how I was doing. "Terrific!" I said. I knew and they knew I was not. However, it was important to keep telling myself I was OK. *Stay positive*, I thought.

I kept the tightly wound scarf on my head. I was hoping it would hold my hair in place until I made it through my appointment. I feared my hair would fall out in front of everyone in the waiting room. I constantly felt my hair and scarf to reassure myself they were still there.

When I saw my oncologist, he was impressed. He asked me how I'd kept my hair. I laughed as I told him I was holding it in place with the scarf. I said it would be gone the next time he saw me.

I went to the infusion room to prepare for my second treatment. I was greeted by the nurses who were my unsung heroes. Every time I entered the room they were pleasant and supportive. They were truly more of my "angels." The nurse accessed my port and began the IV fluids. The numbing cream worked great—I had no pain this time!

I sat in the recliner, watching the drugs drip into my body. I was restless. I saw the lady whom I had met in the waiting room sitting across the way, receiving treatment. Her name was Karen. She was receiving the same treatment I was but was six weeks ahead of me in the treatment plan. I wanted to talk to her about my side effects. I wanted to know more about her side effects and her diagnosis. She had completed her Red Devil Cocktails and started her Taxol treatments. I knew I had just a short time to talk to her because the nausea medicines would soon make me drowsy. She was awake as well, so it was an opportune time for me to go and talk to her. I unplugged my IV companion and rolled it over to her chair. (The IV machine dispensed the drugs and fluids into my body for approximately 3 to 4 hours. When it was unplugged, it was powered by a battery pack so the drugs and fluids could pump continuously without interruption. It was on rollers, which made it easy to navigate to other places such as the restroom. When you are receiving lots of fluids and drugs during the four-hour infusion, you have to be able to take a restroom break!)

Karen must have thought I was nuts rolling my IV machine over to her chair. It was as if I were meeting her for a tea party. (Hey, you have to make the best of every situation and every moment in your life, whether you are in the midst of something good or something bad!) We talked briefly and soon I had to go back to my chair because my "Happy Hour" was starting to take effect. I would see Karen several more times as the weeks passed. She became a "chemo buddy" and one of the best supporters during and after my treatment was completed. We were there for each other for moral support and information. It was nice having someone who could relate to what I was experiencing physically and mentally.

I finished my four-hour treatment and Steve and I went home. Two Red Devil Cocktails completed and two more to go. This was a big mental step for me, knowing I had completed half of this nightmarish treatment. However, two weeks of mental and physical pain remained in front of me. At home, I prepared my large glass of ice water and began pushing the liquids immediately. (I did not want to return to the office again for fluids.) I pushed the fluids hard, but it was tough. I didn't want to drink because I was nauseous, but the ice water felt comforting to my burning throat and stomach. Again, I nestled into the comfy couch to work my way through the mental and physical pain of the chemotherapy treatment.

My whole digestive tract burned and churned, my headache returned, and my eyesight became blurry again. The nausea increased. The drugs made me shake. Again, all I could do was focus on each second until it passed. (The cycle would continue for the next two weeks.)

By the next morning, I was extremely nauseous again and immediately took my two nausea medicines and Phenergan to help get past the wave of sickness. I cat-napped throughout the day until it was time to return for my shot. Again, my good friend Erum picked me up and took me to the doctor's office. The ride made me nauseous and it hurt to talk. Again, I put a scarf on my head to hold my hair in place. My hair was a sorry sight, but I still had some!

I returned home and sat on my comfy couch. The mental and physical pain was building. It was hitting me quicker and harder this round.

Towards the evening, I realized it was time to do something with my hair before I hit the peak of the che-motherapy's churn and burn. I had not washed it for several days. It was falling out faster and in larger clumps, making a mess everywhere I went.

Later that night, I told my kids it was time to remove my hair. I asked Steve to come into my bathroom to shave my head. Though it was upsetting to me, I tried to prepare them for the shock of what I would look like without hair. Clay was visibly upset but Corey acted as if nothing was wrong. I tried to make light of it all, saying that it was only hair. I explained I would still be the same mom but without hair. Clay finally joined Steve and me in the bathroom.

First we cropped the strands of my chin-length hair as short as we could. It was all I could do to stand there and let Steve cut and shave my head. The full torments of the drugs were hitting my body. I had a headache, my vision was blurry, my nervous system was raw, and I was shaking. I was burning from the top of my mouth to the bottom of my stomach. I was weak and could hardly stand while Steve shaved my head. Clay wanted me to save some strands of my hair. He went to get a baggie and we placed a small amount of hair in it. (I believe in Clay's mind he was saving a part of me. It was his way of controlling his fear of losing me.) Steve then shaved my head with the electric razor. It looked like I had a black plastic cap on my head when he finished. Finally, I had a buzz haircut. I cried and laughed at the same time.

I needed to take a shower to wash away the hair sticking to the back of my neck. I crawled under the hot shower to try to wash away the cut hair and the pain, but the latter would not go away. I started shampooing my head. I looked down at my hands. They were black. The short hair left on my head was coming off into my hands every time I rubbed my head. It frightened me at first. I rubbed and rinsed several times. Each time I rubbed my head, my hands were black. I started crying. The black hair kept coming on my hands. It wouldn't quit! I rubbed my head again and again, until there was no more. It was gone. I was bald.

Even though I knew I would lose my hair, the reality shook me. I got out of the shower and looked into the mirror. I felt like a freak. It was as if a total stranger was looking back at me. I did not recognize myself. I was totally detached mentally from my body.

There was no positive thought for me to think of at this point. Just when you think you've reached the lowest point, something like this moves you past that point. I was human. I broke down and sobbed.

I dressed and went to sit on my comfy couch. Corey appeared to be OK with my baldness, but Clay was still somewhat upset. (I could only imagine what this was like for him—or any child—seeing his mother change drastically within the hour. It had to be traumatic for both of my children.) I put a sock hat on my head to help disguise the baldness and to keep my head warm. Clay and I snuggled together on the couch, which comforted both of us. Soon, night was upon us and everyone went to bed except me. I prepared my fluids and melted into the comfy couch for the long haul that lay in front of me. I had to rebuild my mental strength and prepare for the night ahead. This time I knew what to expect: The next 36 to 96 hours were going to be brutal.

Thirty-six hours after the second Red Devil Cocktail treatment, the torturous hell began again. During the thrust of the churn and burn, I started experiencing some thoughts I'd had never experienced in my life. They were thoughts of despair, helplessness, and a beginning of an end. It scared me. I began to spiral down and couldn't stop. I started crying. This was a black hole and I needed to get out of it, but I could not. With God's help, I learned to detach my mind from my body and told myself there would be better thoughts in a few days. At least, I hoped there would be. *Just get by this second*, I told myself.

When I first experienced these thoughts, I was alone in the middle of the night. It scared me. But I soon learned that I would have these thoughts on every Thursday following my treatments—every time. I would enter this mental state again and again. I would prepare myself mentally and wait for it to hit. *Just take it a second at a time*, I told myself. I would do my best to block the thoughts when they began, reminding myself that they were not going to last. At times I would slip and I would begin to panic. I spoke to God. He was there every time. Again, He was there to bridge my seconds together. He always arrived on time. He helped me past the pain until I passed the peak of the drugs churning and burning inside.

I found after each subsequent treatment, I tended to accumulate new side effects while the old side effects became more intense. It was not until I woke up on the 10th day after my second treatment that I felt halfway decent. My good times would start at seconds, then minutes, then half hours, then a couple of consecutive hours. The pain, churn, and burn would sway and cycle. However, I never would return to normal. Each new treatment day started a little worse than where I had been on the previous treatment day. Tomorrow, I would face my third Red Devil Cocktail. I was not looking forward to this. It was rough. But I did not have time to stop. I had to **_March Forth_**. For now, I had completed two of the four Red Devil Cocktail treatments.

22

ANGELS AMONG US

My Third "Red Devil Cocktail" Treatment

On Monday morning, April 23, 2009, I prepared myself for my third Red Devil Cocktail. I was dreading it. Although I was technically halfway through the treatment, I was telling myself I would be 75 percent finished by the end of the day.

It was a beautiful spring morning—sunny, blue skies and warm. The air was filled with birds singing; the smell of spring flowers and new grass lingered in the air. I tried to focus on this pleasant morning, but it was hard. I had four hours before Steve would come home from work to pick me up and take me to the doctor's office for my third treatment.

I needed something to occupy my mind so I wouldn't dwell on the afternoon's treatment or how I felt. I decided to go to the grocery store and pick up a few items. I did not feel well. After buying a few groceries, I stopped at the gas station. As I was filling up my car, a lady approached me.

"Excuse me," she said. "I don't mean to be nosy, but are you going through chemotherapy for breast cancer?"

"Yes," I said. "I _had_ breast cancer and I am going through preventive chemotherapy treatments now."

She talked to me briefly and told me to hang in there. She had gone through the same treatment 10 years earlier and wanted to come over and give me support. I thanked her for her encouragement.

"We are sisters," she said. "Can I give you a hug?" she asked.

"Yes!" I said.

She gave me a hug and then walked to her car and drove away. I don't remember her name, but the simple act of encouragement was what I needed to get by until my appointment. Her gesture lifted me the rest of the day and, most importantly, through my third treatment. She was an angel walking into my life at the right time, when I needed a lift.

Sometimes we have experiences in our lives that we take for granted. I believe we have angels around us ready to help. Many times they offer us simple acts of human kindness. Sometimes we fail to recognize these acts and continue to bemoan our situation, looking at the negative. Again, God arrived right on time for me that day. This lady gave me the spiritual lift I needed to help me through the third treatment. She was a telling example how time and again I received help from my angels.

As I drove home, I realized that I had many angels who walked with me during this experience. I cannot thank them enough other than to dedicate this book to all of them. What an unbelievable group of people who came to help and pray for me and my family. Some were strangers. Some were in the medical field. Some were family and friends. Some were simple acquaintances who became very good friends throughout this journey.

In some small way, I hope I can reach out to those who may not have a support system as I did. I hope I can be there for those who reached out to me if and when they need help. It is so important to remain positive and forward thinking. The village that surrounds you will help encourage and remind you as you go through this crisis. Remember to surround yourself with positive people!

Even the smallest gesture can help someone get through a challenging moment. An e-mail or a phone call can arrive at the most opportune time to help you to the next second. Never underestimate the smallest of tasks when a person is going through a crisis such as cancer treatment.

Debra was another angel. She was a good friend during my treatment. She called me almost every day, bringing me flowers, food, or a book to help me pass my time. She would leave a message on my answering system at times when I was too weak to pick up the phone. But I heard her voice encouraging me to hang in there. I am thankful for her encouragement and pleasant spirit with each call and visit.

Erum was another angel and kind friend. She also called or visited me every other day to make sure I stayed focused on the positive. She helped me get to my appointments and offered encouragement through brief visits. She was the first friend to see me bald and responded with kind ego building words when I needed them the most.

I wish I could list everyone who helped me. Many people helped to transport our sons to and from sports, school, church, and 4-H functions. It became a village of people looking after our kids. Friends and family would encourage me through e-mails and cards. Some brought food and gift baskets for my family. Our church became one big family extending themselves out to us. My friends' churches put me and my family on their prayer lists. I was truly humbled by these experiences. They cared so much for me and my family. Many made sure we did not fall.

The whole experience renewed my faith in people. We hear so much about the negative things in the world that they overtake the positive. We really do have a lot to be thankful for in our lives, especially here in the United States.

I do believe there are angels among us. The group Alabama summed it up best in their song "Angels Among Us." When life gave me troubles and brought me to my knees, someone came along to comfort me and help me, whether it was a stranger or a friend. When the road was dark, God and his angels gave me a ray of hope. They showed up in the strangest places and gave me grace and mercy at the times I needed it. Again, God arrived right on time.

When I came home from the grocery store, I prepared for my third treatment. Again, I packed my jacket, prayer shawl, earphones, and nausea medicine and applied the numbing cream to my port area. Steve arrived home and we left for the doctor's office to complete my third Red Devil Cocktail. Again it was the same ritual: sign in, "How are you doing?", "Terrific", etc. I saw the oncologist and returned to the infusion room for my chemotherapy drugs.

Today will be a good day in the infusion room, I told myself. I would get through this just like the lady who hugged me today and every other woman who had been treated for breast cancer.

I sat in the recliner and waited for the nurses to access my port. I began talking to the lady next to me. She also was a breast cancer survivor. Her name was Tammy and she was beginning the same treatment I was having. She was having her first Red Devil Cocktail. I felt sorry for her because she had no idea what she was about to experience in the next two weeks. No matter how much the nurse tries to prepare you for the side effects, it never comes close to the real thing. We talked briefly, but then my "Happy Hour" began and I fell asleep. Tammy became another angel in my life and my second "chemo buddy."

Tammy and I both had a deep faith in God. Both of us had a strong will to succeed and a need to get through this experience positively. I know that God put us on the same path so that we would meet and help each other through this journey. Each future treatment, I would look forward to seeing her. We would review our progress and make light of our situation. Humor helped both of us. We soon found that the chemotherapy affected us in a lot of the same ways and yet differently as well. I experienced some side effects more strongly than she did and she experienced others more strongly than I did, but for the most part we shared many of the same side effects.

We reinforced the positive, never letting the other fall into the pits much like a soldier would not leave his wounded comrade on the battlefield. It was the beginning of a lasting friendship in which we helped each other through our chemotherapy treatments as well as our recovery. It was as if she was my left side and I was her right side. We developed a solid bond of friendship as we both struggled to complete our treatments. Next to Steve, she was my best supporter during the rest of my chemotherapy infusions. Each week I would look forward to seeing her so we could share our progress. It was great having someone with whom to discuss my side effects or share my questions and concerns. I was thankful that most of her appointments followed mine.

After my infusion was completed, I went home to get my ice water and sit on my comfy couch. Again, I would melt into the couch and mentally and physically prepare for what was lying ahead of me for the next 5 to 6 days.

After experiencing two Red Devil Cocktail treatments, I had noticed a pattern to my side effects:

- **Day—Treatment Day:** Best day to feel good during your treatment cycle. Best part of the day—"Happy Hour," when you receive the antinausea medicines during your treatment. The drugs make you sleep. It is the most restful sleep of the two-week treatment. (I called it my margarita.) After-treatment symptoms: severe headache, nausea, mouth dryness, increasing stomach and digestive tract churning and burning, brownish red urine. Extreme tiredness intensifies.

- **Day 2:** Each one of the above symptoms increases and intensifies. Nausea increases. Brownish red urine decreases. Very little to no appetite. Thirst increases—drink, drink, and drink *lots* of liquids. Take antinausea medicines. Report back to doctor's office for white blood cell count booster shot. Did I mention the drugs intensify all symptoms and nausea increases?! The sustained nightmarish hours begin towards the evening and continue for the next 3 to 4 days.
- **Days 3-6**: Chemotherapy drugs are at full strength. Take final antinausea medicines. The churn and burn is extreme. The nightmare continues. The torch burns from my mouth to my bottom. Hemorrhoids, diarrhea, mouth sores, headache, blurry vision, and light-headedness continue. My body feels raw and terrible at all hours. Extreme nausea makes it hard to eat or drink. I feel as if I could vomit bleach. It is impossible to talk to people.
- **Days 4 and 5:** Drugs still at full strength and intensity. Salt cravings and foot cramps begin. Light-headedness continues. Tingling and numbness in the bottoms of feet intensify. It is pure hell! Mental

and physical pain! Despairing thoughts begin and collide with the pain. Thoughts of dying surge in my mind. Exhaustion. Sleeping is almost impossible because you feel so bad and your body is in turmoil. I recline flaccidly on the couch until a reprieve comes. These 48 hours become the expansive seconds that I walk with God.

- **Days 6 and 7:** Reprieve begins. Some bright spots start to surface. The tornado has passed and the sun shines a little. Smaller headache. Still have light-headedness, eyes still somewhat blurry. Challenging to read and comprehend. Able to sit up on the couch. Able to read at computer and open mail. Appetite starts to return. Exhaustion replaces the tiredness. Nervous system makes me shake. Extremely sick to the stomach. Churn and burn continues. Again, it feels like I could vomit bleach.

- **Day 8:** Able to write e-mail but head continues to feel like it is being squeezed. Vision still somewhat blurry. Feel total disconnect from my body. Diarrhea. Feel like making calls and talking a little. Head feels like it is disconnected. Appetite returns a little. Feel a little better but still sick. Inside of mouth on fire.

- **Day 9:** Half of my day feels "good" and half feels "bad." Difficult to drink fluids. Throat red. Major sores in mouth and back of throat. Nausea decreases, now feels like a bad case of morning sickness.

- **Day 10:** Begin to sleep better. Able to run one

errand. Very light housework possible. Exhaustion.

- **Days 12-14:** Can accomplish some things if I rest most of the day. General malaise, nausea, and exhaustion. Able to take a small walk.
- **Day 15:** I get to take another treatment and experience all these symptoms again at a greater degree of pain, burning, and nausea.

March Forth! **Amen!**

23
FEEL THE BURN

My Final "Red Devil Cocktail" Treatment

After completing my third Red Devil Cocktail, I could tell that the treatments were hitting me harder and that the bad times were lasting longer and my swings toward recovery were getting shorter. I simply felt terrible after the third treatment. All of my bodily systems were deteriorating after each treatment. My side effects were stronger and more prolonged: more nausea, exhaustion, skin dryness, eye dryness, acid reflux, and more blisters in the mouth, throat, stomach and digestive tract. I had constant burning in these areas. I had acid reflux in the extreme. When I burped, the acid would enter my mouth. My stomach was bloated. I again felt as if I could vomit bleach. I was also experiencing "Chemo brain." (I describe Chemo brain as an absence of thinking. The brain seems to fill with air. Thoughts stop circulating. Blank stares are common!)

At the end of my treatment week was Easter. I had bought a ham the previous week in hopes of feeling good enough to make a simple Easter dinner. I am not sure what I was thinking when I did this because I soon found I was only kidding myself. The effort it took to cook as well as the smell of cooking made me nauseous and exhausted. Besides, I had no appetite. I placed the ham in the freezer for another time.

Steve, Corey, and Clay went to our church for Easter services and breakfast. I stayed home and watched Easter services on television. When it was time for my family to return home, I got out of bed. I had bought some candy a few days earlier, towards the end of my recovery week. I went outside and placed it in the yard for an Easter egg hunt for old time's sake. I walked to the end of the yard, throwing the candy as I went, and then walked back, nauseated and exhausted. I was trying to keep our traditions alive, but it was hard. I went back to bed shortly after everyone came home from church. Later I had a small appetite and Steve went to Cracker Barrel and bought our family some comfort food. This was our Easter dinner.

After my third treatment, during my recovery week, I decided to mop my floor. I felt like I needed to do something constructive and productive. I was so sick of being sick! Several people said they would mop the floor for me but I needed to gain some independence and feel less sick and helpless. I got a bucket of water and a towel and got on my hands and knees. I began mopping the large 18" x 18" square tiles in my kitchen. My arm was still hurting from the mastectomy. I thought maybe using it would help it. The mopping was exhausting.

First I mopped four squares, then I slept two hours.

When I awoke, I mopped a couple more squares. Again, I was exhausted and napped some more. I continued all day until I had a 10' x 14' area of my floor completed. I felt like I had accomplished something, and my arm felt better after mopping with it.

I was beginning to think the nerve endings in my arm were transmitting false pain to my brain. Maybe I needed to reboot the signals from my arm to my brain just as I sometimes reboot my computer to clear its jammed software. Apparently, mopping was the best medicine for the whole mastectomy site and my arm. The arm felt better after working the towel on the floor. In the future, I tried to work the arm as much as I could. It had been eight weeks since my surgery. I needed to concentrate on healing this site in addition to surviving the chemotherapy treatments.

During the weekend before my fourth and final Red Devil Cocktail, it was apparent I was not improving physically like I had after the previous treatments. I simply felt better lying down. Sunday night before my final treatment, I became very nauseous. As I was lying down, I thought, *Tomorrow will be my last Red Devil Cocktail. Thank God!*

On Monday morning, May 4, 2009, I walked into the doctor's office for my final Red Devil Cocktail. After the staff made sure my lab results were normal, I walked into the infusion room to begin treatment. After a torturous six weeks, I had three treatments down and one to go before I completed this drug regimen. I was nauseous during my doctor's appointment and nauseous as they started my final treatment.

When I finished my treatment, Steve and I drove home. I thought I was going to throw up in the car. I was absolutely sick. At home, I slid onto my comfy couch. This time I sat on the couch and fell over on my side, keeping my feet on the floor. I did not have the energy to move. I was extremely nauseous. The treatments had never hit me this hard so early after the infusion. It was the beginning of a very long two weeks.

The burning and churning in my digestive tract and nauseous state steadily increased through the night. In my previous treatments, this surge usually arrived around the 48th hour and lasted through the sixth day before my reprieve started. *My God,* I thought: *if I feel this bad now, what will I feel like at the 48th hour?* I had a five-gallon bucket sitting beside me. I was too weak to make it to the bathroom if the urge to vomit came. I thought if I started to vomit, I would not stop. By early morning, as the sun began to rise, the drugs were at full strength inside my body. I could not move on the couch. I remember Steve coming over to look at me and ask if I was OK. It was all I could do to answer: "My God, I am so sick!"

My friend Erum came later to take me to the doctor's office for my white blood cell booster shot. I was so weak I could hardly get into the vehicle. It hurt to talk. Trying to talk took away my focus on ignoring the pain and nausea. Therefore, I didn't talk.

If I used what energy I had for other things, I had no energy to fight the pain and nausea. I had to conserve what energy I had to focus past the pain. This was why it was hard to have visitors during the second through sixth days of this treatment. When we arrived at the infusion room, the nurse gave me my booster shot and told me to go home and take a Phenergan pill. I went home immediately and took one pill. I slept for 12 hours straight. I don't think I moved during those 12 hours.

For the next five days and nights, my body was in full torment from the drugs. I experienced the churn and burn and nausea like never before in my life. This treatment simply knocked me out. I lay on the couch for the next five days, flat on my back. I could not move. On the sixth day after my treatment, I was finally able to sit up. I found I had several blisters where my lips met. Since the drugs destroy all fast-growing cells, including healthy ones, they simply burn you up from your lips all the way through to your bottom. My insides hurt. It felt like a blowtorch from my lips to my bottom. It hurt my insides for my bowels to move. It felt like acid sloshing inside my stomach. Again, I felt like I could vomit bleach.

Today, I had a new side effect. I could taste blood. Blisters ran rampant in my mouth. My taste buds were shot. If I was going to eat something, it had to be soft foods. It felt like I was going to tear a hole in my digestive tract when I swallowed food. I concentrated on eating cold soups because warm soup would irritate the blisters in my digestive tract. Ice cream was the best thing going—especially a Frosty from Wendy's.

The following Sunday was Mother's Day. I wanted to do something. I called my dad and told him I would try to come and pick him up later in the afternoon for ice cream. I rested all day so I could make the trip to my dad's. He lived approximately 20 minutes from my home. Dad and my family went to the Tastee Freeze Ice Cream Shop and had ice cream for Mother's Day. It was the only thing I did all day and it was the first thing that had tasted good all week. The cold, creamy cone was a blessing on my throat and stomach. I had another one.

We took Dad back and returned home. The total trip had taken two hours. I was exhausted. I slept the rest of the night. Towards the end of the eighth day after my treatment week, I began to have a small appetite. I was restless and nauseated for the rest of my recovery week. By the weekend before my next treatment, I was able to do a few chores. It was tough but I ***Marched Forth.***

24
THE POWER OF PRAYER

I believe in God and I believe in the power of prayer. I am grateful and thankful that God is in my life and walks with me daily. I have felt His power and presence throughout my life and this journey. I felt the healing prayers that many people prayed for me. Most of all, I felt God's presence in the wee hours of the night when I was by myself feeling isolated, nauseous, and in pain.

I believe in prayer and the goodness it can bring in one's life. I have seen and felt its work throughout my life. One of the most telling times was during my mom's last hours of life. Mom lay in her hospice bed. We were keeping a vigil over her and waiting for her to pass. She had become unresponsive. I hated seeing her suffer. She had been given morphine to help her through the final stage of passing. I could hardly stand it. I went to the bathroom and prayed:

> "Dear God: I don't know if it is right for me
> to pray this, but please take her. Please don't
> let her suffer anymore."

When I finished my prayer, I heard my sister Michele speaking to my mom. My mom had spoken to Michele as soon as I'd completed my prayer!

It had been several hours since my mom had spoken. Suddenly, she talked. I asked my sister what Mom had said. Michele heard her say she was going to see her mother and she was ready to go to heaven. I was somewhat taken aback at first that Mom had responded immediately following my prayer. It gave me chills. I felt the power of that prayer being answered. Time moved forward. We continued our vigil.

After several hours, I began to doubt my prayer had been answered. I started questioning whether it was a coincidence. Did God really hear and answer my prayer, or did I just want to think He did? Mom continued to be unresponsive after uttering those few words earlier in the day. Was it a coincidence? Again, I went to the bathroom and prayed:

> "God, I truly believe in you. I don't want to think Mom's answer was a coincidence. I am not sure if it is correct to ask You to take her to heaven. I am sorry if it isn't but I cannot stand to see her suffering and struggling any more. Can you please take Mom to heaven?"

Again, immediately after I completed the prayer, I heard my sister say something to my mom. Again, I asked my sister what happened. Again, my mom had spoken. Again, she'd said that she was ready to go to heaven. This was no coincidence. God was hearing my prayers.

God heard me the first and the second time I prayed. He answered my prayers when Mom responded with those few words—twice. My mom had not spoken all day except for those two responses following my prayers. God was hearing me and He _was_ at my Mom's side. There was no doubting.

It was getting late at Mom's home and she was show-ing signs of passing sooner rather than later. I decided to go home and get a few hours of sleep in my own bed and then return in the morning. But more importantly, I had to go home and tell my small children that their grandma was very, very sick. They knew Grandma had a disease called cancer and it was making her sicker every day. I had kept my answers to their questions very basic throughout the past two years. I did not give them all the information about Mom but I did not mislead them either. I concentrated on positive moments while they were around their grandma.

As I tucked my children into bed for the night, we again said our prayers. I again talked about Grandma and emphasized how very sick she was. We prayed for her and others who were sick. After several questions, Corey asked point-blank, "Is she going to die, Mom?" I paused and thought. I could not lie to him or Clay. It was the truth. She was going to die. I was going to hurt my children when I answered that question. There was only one answer, and it was "yes."

My response opened several more questions and solutions to help Grandma live. However, I explained only
God knows the real reasons and He needs Grandma at
this time more than we need her. She will meet Jesus. She
will see her mother, father, siblings and friends who have
also passed. It will be a happy occasion for her when she
goes to heaven soon. When she dies, God will take care
of her and she will no longer be in pain. We will need to
continue to make our lives positive and productive because that would make Grandma proud. We will miss
her but someday we will all see Grandma again. She will
always be a part of us and who we are.

I tucked my children into bed and kissed them good-
night. It was a heavy load for them to carry. As a mother,
I would need to comfort them as much as I could. I came
downstairs and realized I needed to digest the fact that
I was about to lose my mother to that dreadful disease
called cancer.

Children can ask some of the most challenging questions. When I told my children that Grandma was going
to die, it led to all kinds of questions about life in general.
I did my best to answer these questions. It was interesting to listen to their perspective. I was able to answer
their questions and handle Mom's situation because of
my faith and beliefs.

Children are affected differently by the incidents in
their lives. Parents are faced with challenging questions
because of these incidents. As a parent, I faced these
questions sooner than I wanted to. However, I was extremely fortunate to have parents who taught me about

faith and belief in God. I have taught my children as well.

My son Clay asked me one of those challenging questions as a child. "Why doesn't God answer me when I pray, Mom? I am listening but I cannot hear him and he doesn't answer me back. How do I know he is there and hears me?" he asked me one day.

This was a tough question. But my response was simple. "God hears you, son. Most times he answers you indirectly." I explained that God is like the wind or air that surrounds us. We cannot actually see the wind, air, or God. But they are there. When the wind blows, it moves the leaves in the trees or the blades of grass on our lawn. The air sends the smell of the fresh-baked cookies to our noses. We can see, hear, smell, and feel the effects of the wind and the air. God moves in much the same way. Sometimes we miss His answers because we are not watching, listening, or feeling as perceptively as we should be. Sometimes He answers us when we are helped by a friend in our time of need. God never leaves us.

He answered my prayers for Mom. I had begun to doubt His first answer. But I prayed again, he answered me again through my mother. For me, I cannot deny that the wind exists any more than I can deny God exists.

Life brings us results. Sometimes we don't like the results. The results are not what we want. This can make us angry. Sometimes people don't get what they want in life and become angry at God and blame Him. Some people turn away from God during these crises; sometimes these crises make people turn to God. The one thought we all need to remember is this: Even though we may turn away from God, God never turns away from us.

Sometimes we question the results we have in life. For example, some may ask, "Why did God give me cancer?" I do not believe God gave me cancer. What I do believe is God gave me free will to choose. Maybe my choices or others' choices affected my body, making it susceptible to cancer. I do not know. I can't see God's big picture. However, I do know that God has a plan for me. As a human being, I sometimes do not understand the plan. This can make things complicated because God gives us free will to choose.

When we have free will, we can make choices that affect us. We as humans cannot control choices that other people make. However, we can control our thoughts and try to strive for what God wants us to do for our fellow man. Human nature is flawed; therefore some things happen in life that as humans we wish did not happen. We are not perfect so we just have to do the best that we can each day. Sometimes when we cannot do our best, we have strangers, friends, family (all angels), and a higher being to help us through.

As far as God answering my child when he prays, God may answer him in many different ways. Maybe the answer comes from me or an action by another. Maybe God answers us directly but we are not listening. It is important for all of us to listen carefully and help our fellow man.

Faith makes weak people strong. Faith in God makes me stronger. God shapes us and molds us through our life experiences. Some of us listen and learn from them and some do not. He teaches us so we may teach others as we face life's challenging moments. Some day we will all understand why things happen. In the meantime, God will take care of you and me.

Therefore with that in mind, I continued to **_March Forth_** as positively as I could on my journey. It was hard. But tough times build character. Apparently God thought I needed more character. I never doubted Him through my journey. He was there for me when I physically and mentally needed Him. When my physical and mental weaknesses collided, God carried me.

Thus, many times during this journey, whether in the middle of the day or the wee hours of the night, I talked to God. I prayed for healing. I prayed for a cure. I prayed for others who were battling this disease. I prayed for those who were having difficult times. I prayed for my family and friends who were praying for _me._ I gave thanks for all He had given me. Each night I would finish my prayer by asking God to allow me to receive the positive healing and comfort that many were praying for me. Each time after this request, I had an indescrible physical feeling travel through my body. I felt it travel from my head to my toes. The power of positive prayer was working for me. I felt it.

I was thankful my situation was survivable. I tried to stay positive. It was not easy, and I cried many times.

But I was going to get through this. I knew I had to stay mentally positive. This was my job. God would take care of the rest. I trusted Him. I was at His mercy. I would get through this journey with Him. Thanks be to God! *__March Forth__*!

25

TAXOL-12 TREATMENTS AND COUNTING

At the end of the recovery week from my final Red Devil Cocktail, I realized I did not have a prescription for antinausea drugs for my next treatment. I was scheduled to begin my Taxol treatments on Monday, May 23, 2009. I called the nurse and requested the prescriptions. She explained I would not need it. I didn't understand. One of the side effects of Taxol was nausea. "Why wouldn't I take antinausea medicines?" I asked. She explained that Taxol was not as tough as the Red Devil Cocktail. *OK*, I thought. But I was not convinced.

I had recently completed the most nauseous period in my life and I was going in for 12 more treatments without antinausea medicines!? Whoa!!! My anxiety level began to climb. Furthermore, the Taxol treatments were separated by only one week of recovery not two, like the Red Devil Cocktails had been. I was not going to have a second week to recover. This concerned me, to put it mildly.

Two weeks following my fourth Red Devil Cocktail, I went to the oncologist's office to have my first Taxol treatment. When I arrived for my appointment, it was the same ritual again: Sign in, "How're you doing?,"

"Terrific," pay the co-pay, draw my blood for the CBC, etc. When I saw the oncologist, I explained how debilitating the chemotherapy had been for me the past two weeks. He stated that is why only four "devil" treatments are given in succession. Any more and the chemotherapy would take a person past the edge. (Amen, brother!)

We discussed the side effects and dosing procedure of the Taxol and the results of my CBC. Although some of my blood counts were lower than any previous lab results, I was within the parameters that allowed me to begin the new chemotherapy treatment. I proceeded to the infusion area to receive my first Taxol treatment.

Taxol has a tendency to cause an allergic reaction. Thus, I was watched extremely closely when I received my first dose. The nurses administered medicines to prevent an allergic reaction and to prevent stomach upset. I was also given steroids to help with these side effects. By the time the Taxol drug was entering my body, my "Happy Hour" was in full swing. My eyelids were heavy and my words slurred. Again, I succumbed to my "expensive margarita." No matter how hard I tried to stay awake, I went to sleep. It was always the most restful sleep of my week.

As soon as I finished my treatment, I could hardly wait to get out of the building. I walked as fast as I could to get to the car. My legs were very heavy. They felt like I had 100-pound weights on them. It was hard for my legs to keep up with my mind. When I got home, I went to my security blanket—my comfy couch. I waited for the freight train to hit me like it did after the Red Devil

Cocktails. But, it did not. I slept most of the evening and night. I was wiped out.

When the next morning came, I woke up and sent my kids off to school. Where was the freight train? It had not arrived. I felt "good" compared to after the Red Devil Cocktail. I had a small appetite on the day following treatment! I was forewarned that most patients put on weight with this treatment. If I felt this "good" after each treatment, I could see why I would put on weight, too! I continued to watch my diet and eat as healthily as I could.

Forty-eight hours after the treatment, I still felt decent compared to after the Red Devil Cocktails. My stomach continued to burn but not nearly to the degree it had following the Red Devil Cocktails. Some of my symptoms were swollen eyes, burning nose, mild nausea, burning in my stomach, and tingling in my hands and feet. My nasal passages were extremely dry. I also had a small headache.

Towards the end of the third day following my initial Taxol treatment, my nausea increased, but it was manageable. My mouth and stomach continued to burn, but nothing like the churn and burn following the Red Devil Cocktail. Even though I was exhausted, I fixed dinner that evening. I was able to walk, but I had to stop and rest three times.

On the fourth day, sores continued to develop around my gums. These mouth sores continued to increase after each treatment. I nursed them with salt water, hydrogen peroxide, and a prescription called Martha's Magic Mouthwash.

My stomach began to bloat. Towards the evening, I felt as if I had to urinate but couldn't. This bloating would continue through the very last Taxol treatment.

On the fifth, sixth, and seventh day following my initial Taxol treatment, I was slowly but surely feeling better. I also was able to drive short distances.

My Taxol treatments continued each week. My side effects increased and persisted after each treatment. Bloating, swelling, and weight gain gradually increased. The numbness in my hands, lower legs, and feet was greater after each treatment. My skin was *very* dry and sensitive and it hurt for anything to touch it. I had no oil in my glands. I developed nosebleeds. My nervous system felt raw, and I would shake uncontrollably at times. Indescribable exhaustion and tiredness continued.

My body hurt all over—especially my muscles. It felt as if I had exercised to the max and my muscles were filled with lactic acid. It felt as if a Mack truck had driven over me several times. This ache would continue to worsen after each Taxol treatment. The pain actually increased after my treatments ended! (It began to improve approximately 11 months out from the end of my last treatment.)

Like clockwork, four days after my treatment I would enter a depression. I would despair, sometimes crying uncontrollably, thinking that I was going to die. Finally, I just let myself cry when these feelings overtook me. In my mind, I knew most of these dark thoughts would lift after the 48-hour period.

One night I awoke while experiencing this depression

stage during my treatment week. I began crying. I awakened Steve because I was sobbing loudly. He asked, "What's the matter?" I said, "I am going to die." He said, "No you're not! You are going to be OK!" After hearing those words, I *was* OK. I stopped crying and went to sleep.

It is so important for your friends and family to remind you that things are going well and you are going to be OK. The drugs temporarily rob you of your logic and you need to be reminded of the simplest things. The mental and physical grind of the treatment constantly challenge your strength and your psyche. It was very tough when the mental and physical grind would peak at the same time. I knew it was important to remain positive and mentally strong. I had to endure the pain or quit. I chose not to quit. During this process, it was also important to stay away from negative people.

It was OK to cry. However, every time I started to cry, I stopped, so I could remain strong. I told myself I could not let myself sink. I was afraid if I started crying I would not have the strength to build my mental wall again to block the pain and sickness the chemotherapy caused. I didn't want to expend my energy rebuilding that mental wall I'd constructed to fight the pain and sickness. Therefore, when I cried it was for short bouts then I forced myself back to focusing on going forward again.

As my treatments continued, I became more light-headed. I started having nosebleeds regularly. I continued to feel more exhausted; my sleep was broken, which added to my exhaustion. Sometimes I slept well but most times I did not.

After my fifth Taxol treatment, I again felt "good", even somewhat euphoric. As a result, I did more things around the house. However, I paid a heavy price for my extra activities. I immediately felt bad following my sixth treatment and did not recover before the seventh treatment began.

After my sixth Taxol treatment, my lab results showed my red and white blood cell counts were lower than they had been at any time throughout my treatment. I felt more tired and exhausted than ever before, if that was possible. Each treatment was slowly robbing me of my health and strength.

Some people need blood transfusions during treatments because some blood counts are outside of the CBC parameters. Others need to postpone treatments until their CBC results fall within the parameters. The labwork taken before each doctor's visit is used to monitor these complete blood counts. Again, the CBC is a deciding factor before allowing treatment.

After my sixth Taxol treatment, I started having a lot of nosebleeds. Sometimes I would have several per day. The insides of my nostrils were extremely dry. I had no fluids to moisten the air passages. I also did not have any hair lining my nostrils. (The Red Devil Cocktail doesn't just cause the hair on your head to fall out!) It hurt to breathe. It felt as if a torch was burning a hole through my nostrils with every breath. I used saline nose spray several times a day to help with the dryness.

After several nosebleeds in one day, I called the oncology nurse. The doctor requested a culture test to check for other possible problems in my nose. The culture was benign. I then decided to look inside my nose with a penlight. I could not believe what I saw! It looked as if a meat grinder had sliced through each side of my nasal passages. They were full of scabs and cuts. The chemotherapy had literally destroyed my air passages. (The nostrils contain fast-growing cells. Chemotherapy destroys all fast-growing cells, good ones and bad ones.) Thus, my nasal passages were "chewed up." *If my nose looked this bad, what did my digestive tract look like?* I shuddered at these thoughts.

I searched on the Internet for a solution to help heal my nasal passages. (You have to be careful about placing certain creams inside the nostrils because they can harm the lungs. For example, petroleum jelly can harm the lungs.) I found one lady had used an antibiotic cream that contained bacitracin. I had an over-the-counter cream that contained bacitracin, so I started applying small amounts inside my nostrils. It moistened the inside of my nose and the bacitracin helped heal some of the sores. The cream was not recommended for use inside the nasal passages, but I was desperate at that point. My nasal passages were very damaged inside; they could not recover because of my weekly Taxol treatments. And they were only going to get worse. My nasal passages would not start to heal until I stopped the Taxol treatments altogether.

The day before my seventh Taxol treatment, I went

to church for the first time in four months. I attended a church dinner for our retiring minister. I was glad I felt like attending; however, it was extremely exhausting for me. I came home, intending to take a nap, and slept for four hours. I woke up briefly after my nap and went back to bed. I slept until early morning the next day.

This was one of the most frustrating things I went through during the Taxol treatments. I felt better than after the Red Devil Cocktail treatments, but I was too exhausted to attend social events. What little energy I had, was quickly depleted. Talking depleted my energy even faster. I would often return home and sit on my comfy couch. The couch became my refuge where I could recharge my batteries in order to do something else. Those were some long days. I would have to recharge several times a day, depending on the demands placed on my time and energy. I was so limited as to what I could do in a day! This created an isolation issue for me, because I could not socialize.

As I continued my Taxol treatments, I found I was getting more nauseous from the fluids given to me during my infusions. I could taste some of the medicines as they entered my body. I remember my good friend, Joe Clark, told me to take some lemon drops to prevent seasickness when I went on a cruise. He told me the marines used them when they were being transported on warships during World War II. Therefore, I bought some lemon drops to suck on during my treatments. This helped my nausea tremendously. I offered lemon drops to others beside me while I was taking my treatments. I began using lemon drops during the recovery week as well, whenever I became nauseous.

After my seventh Taxol treatment, I felt terrible. I felt horrible all week. Somehow I thought since I had done so well the week before that I would do well after this treatment, but no such luck. I continued to have nose-bleeds and my stomach continued to hurt and bloat. The numbness in my feet was increasing and causing balance problems. My mouth and throat were on fire. I was having heart palpitations again. My fingernails were turning yellow and starting to die. My white blood cell count was dropping. I felt sharp, shooting pains in my right breast.

Although my symptoms were gradually worsening, I had a ray of sunshine: My hair began to grow. I am not sure what color it was. The fuzz was either blonde or white. I optimistically convinced myself it was blonde. I did not want to be white or gray headed.

As my Taxol treatments continued, every large and small muscle in my body hurt. It was painful to move. I struggled to move from a sitting position to a standing position. My legs would shake. It hurt to touch any part of my body. My muscles ached and weakened more after each infusion. The Mack truck was now running over me continuously. Simply stated, my body—especially my muscles—hurt like crazy.

Each week I set small goals to survive the chemo-therapy regimen. For example, after three treatments I told myself I had completed 25 percent of my treatments; after the fourth treatment I had completed 33 percent; after the sixth I had 50 percent, and so on. I had to focus on small, tangible goals each day, each hour, each minute, and sometimes each second to manage the treatments. When I became overwhelmed with the process, I reminded myself that each second I endured brought me closer to completing the treatment. For the next several weeks I continued to count down my weekly Taxol treatments using small achievable goals. I was _Marching_ slowly _Forth._

26

"CHEMO BRAIN"

Fog

Chemotherapy travels throughout the body via the bloodstream. It destroys all fast-growing cells in the body without distinguishing between healthy cells and diseased cells. It kills <u>all</u> fast growing cells. When you undergo chemotherapy, you hope it kills all the bad cells and leaves enough good cells to allow you to function and recover.

Each week the chemotherapy drugs were damaging my body's systems. The side effects were more prolonged and harsher after each treatment. In addition to the side effects mentioned in the previous chapters, I was now experiencing "chemo fog" or "chemo brain" full throttle.

Chemo brain is a condition where the chemotherapy drugs impede the memory. After several chemotherapy treatments, my brain began to struggle. I could not answer simple questions or make simple decisions. I could not remember things that I should remember, such as names and places. At times, Steve would ask me to make a choice between two things and I simply could not. My brain was stagnant.

I struggled to pull the words from my brain and transfer them to my mouth to speak. The information would bluntly stop circulating in my brain. I compared it to a big pipe flowing with water and a knife gate suddenly dropping and stopping the water's flow. As I became more exhausted and tired, the fog became stronger.

I had difficulty concentrating on the simplest of tasks. I could form the thoughts and words in my head, but I physically could not make them come out of my mouth. My mind was totally blanking on names and familiar places. I could not add simple numbers. I could not focus on making logical decisions. The fog would leave me with a blank stare, searching for words and answers as I tried to transfer my thoughts from my brain to my mouth.

"Chemo brain" is not comparable to the simple forgetfulness we experience as we age—for example, walking into a room and forgetting why you came into the room. You know you are going to get something but just can't remember what it is. Your mind cycles over several thoughts, trying to remember why you came into the room. You may or may not remember. Sometimes you start a different task and forget about the task you came in the room to do.

With chemo brain, you walk into the room and don't recognize the room and briefly wonder what house you are in! Things began to look foreign and unrecognizable for split seconds. Your mind does not cycle several thoughts: It stops. No thoughts circulate. When your

mind stops, you are stuck in the few seconds of not rec-
ognizing the room.

Chemo brain is like dumping a large puzzle on the
floor. You logically find two puzzle pieces that fit together, and then your thought process stops. The next logical
step is to put the two puzzle pieces together. However,
with chemo brain, you can't because your brain has
stopped functioning. You have to wait for the brain
waves to start flowing again. Sometimes they start, but
most times, they don't. One's precious energy is spent
trying to remove the knife gate so the water will flow
again. The process of reconnecting and reestablishing
flow is mentally exhausting. And as my chemotherapy
treatment progressed, the fog became worse.

One day I received a get well card from a lady at our
church. I read the card and did not recognize the name.
I could not put a face to it. I had known this lady very
well before chemotherapy. When Steve came home from
work, I asked him about the card. He tried to explain
to me who the lady was. I could not figure it out and
thought about it the rest of the evening. It upset me that
I could not remember.

When I was in public, I began to feel more insecure
about my memory. I didn't know if I would have a glitch
with someone I should know. I began holding on to Steve's
arm for physical as well as mental support. This gesture
would settle me if the anxiety and forgetfulness began.
Again, this fog continued to worsen after each treatment.

One day, Steve and I went shopping. He was driving.
We came to the exit of a well-known store. It was one

of the most highly traveled crossroads in the area. I had driven on those streets many times. I looked both ways and said, "I know where I am. I know if we turn right, we can get home. But I don't recognize anything past this point where we are sitting at this exit." I was lost. My mind could not process another thought other than that we were sitting at the crossroad. At this point, I could not have found my way home.

These blank incidences would happen repeatedly. Again, the more they started happening, the more I began to feel insecure. Sometimes it was frightening because I would have blank flashes as much as six to eight months after my chemotherapy stopped. They could happen at any time.

The chemo brain prevented me from multitasking. It took a lot of energy and thought to perform a simple task. Before the chemotherapy, I was a great multitasker, but now, it became a challenge. Trying to tackle one task at a time and succeeding with it was an all-day affair during my recovery and healing process. For example, the simple pleasure of having holiday meals and visitors overwhelmed me. It made me a nervous wreck. I wanted to stop whatever I was doing and wring my hands. This was something I had enjoyed. But now, it became a challenge, especially after my treatments ended.

It would be over a full year before the chemo brain would clear. As I healed and recovered my mind continued to heal. Although fatigue still affects my concentration, my brain continues to heal and return to its normal function.

27

SURVIVAL OF THE FITNESS

One of my favorite things to do was exercise. I didn't necessarily enjoy motivating myself to exercise, but I did enjoy the health and fitness benefits after exercising. Before I had my mastectomy, I exercised on my treadmill, using an incline. I walked approximately 45 minutes four to five times per week. I also lifted weights two to three times per week. Occasionally, I would mix yoga into my routine. I enjoyed being fit. My doctor advised me to continue to exercise during my chemotherapy. (That was easier said than done!)

After my mastectomy, my exercise regimen was put on hold. Any attempts at fitness were limited because of my surgical site. I also felt lousy after the mastectomy. Thirteen days after my mastectomy, I went in for my port surgery. Three days after my port surgery, I was taking my first chemotherapy treatment. Thus, in 17 days, I had two surgeries and a round of chemotherapy. Needless to say, my body was grounded from all the cuts and infusions.

During the Red Devil Cocktail phase, I decided I would try to do some exercise. I thought movement would help my mastectomy site heal and also improve my overall physical and mental well-being. I wanted to be more independent of the couch. The problem I was facing was that I could only attempt exercise during my recovery week. It was simply impossible to do anything during the infusion or treatment week.

I tried yoga and found it hard to do. When I reached for the ceiling and breathed in, I became light-headed. When I bent over to touch my toes, I would black out. After trying unsuccessfully several different times to do the stretches, I stopped. It was impossible for me to do any kind of yoga movements without becoming light-headed or blacking out. I had to go to plan B.

I had to get my arm and shoulder near the mastectomy site moving. I did not want to get the frozen shoulder that many women get after their mastectomies. I started stretching the shoulder while lying on the floor or in bed. I could do these stretches and exercises lying down, but not standing up. Again, if I stood up and stretched, I would black out.

Next I tried the treadmill. I tried going as slowly as I could on the treadmill without causing the machine to literally stop. If I could manage 10 minutes, I felt like I was succeeding. Again, I could only try this during my recovery week because I was just too sick during the infusion week. However, after a few Red Devil Cocktails, this too became too demanding. I stopped using the treadmill.

Finally, I tried to make it simple. I decided I would walk around my house. Towards the end of my Red Devil Cocktail infusion week, I went outside and walked a lap around my house. I tried to do this five times. Sometimes I made it and sometimes I didn't. Exercise was challenging; I just had to drop my goals to meet them. I tried to keep moving.

It was disappointing that I couldn't really exercise. I felt my fitness diminishing with each passing day during my treatments. I went from 45 minutes on an inclined treadmill to five small laps around my house. Plainly, I was struggling to achieve fitness during my survival.

After I completed the Red Devil Cocktail and started the Taxol infusions, I was able to begin my exercise regimen again. For the first time, I was able to lift my weights. It had been two months since my mastectomy. I tried not to pamper the mastectomy side. I wanted to strengthen my whole body. I also was able to walk almost two miles most days. Sometimes I would have to rest while walking, but it was important for me to keep moving and _finish_. I still could not do yoga because I would black out whenever I bent over to touch my toes.

Some days it was impossible to do anything. I told myself that was OK. I tried not to be too hard on myself. However, it was important to keep moving or _**Marching Forth.**_

28

RUNNING ON EMPTY

As I continued with my weekly Taxol treatments, I was feeling worse each succeeding week, with very little turnaround time for recovery. The cumulative effect of the Taxol treatments was taking its toll on my whole body.

I was now approaching my 10th Taxol treatment. I tried to look for the positives. I only had to endure one more month of treatments. August (my completion month) was in sight.

Each of my side effects was getting worse. I was losing more sensation from my knees to my feet after each treatment. My body was beginning to hold more fluid. My weight was increasing. I began experiencing more heart palpitations. My nosebleeds continued; my nausea increased. White blisters began appearing next to the red blisters in my throat. My blood sugar started to rise. My sleep was not restful. My blood pressure was starting to increase. My stomach continued to burn. My skin was drier than leather. Even my eyes were dry: My body was like a desert, starved of water.

It was painful to eat solids. As I swallowed, it felt as

if the food was tearing my stomach as it passed through. The pain felt comparable to having a third-degree sunburn and having someone rub the sunburn.

On the morning of my 10th Taxol treatment, I finally made it to a physical therapist for the arm pain I had been experiencing since my mastectomy. As usual, I scheduled my appointment on the morning before my chemotherapy infusion. (It was always my strongest and most rested day.) I was so grateful that the therapist was able to manipulate the fascia in my arm and wrist and relieve some of the pain. Finally, I had some relief! I was concerned that I was going to have to live with the pain forever. (After a few more visits, my arm and wrist were mobile again.)

The physical therapist also fitted my arm for a lymphedema sleeve. The elastic sleeve would prevent my arm from swelling caused by lymph fluid accumulating during exercise. (Again, the more lymph nodes that are removed during the mastectomy, the more the lymphatic system is compromised.)

After the physical therapy visit, I went to take my 10th Taxol treatment. I felt terrible. I was totally out of sync. I struggled mentally to overcome the physical dysfunction I felt. It was hard to block out the thought of how much worse I was going to feel tomorrow, after the day's treatment. I was struggling physically and mentally.

After completing my ritual at the doctor's office, I entered the infusion room to receive my treatment. My first chemo buddy Karen (an angel) surprised me with a visit. She came to cheer me through this appointment. A few minutes later, my other chemo buddy Tammy (another angel) arrived for her infusion. All three of us joked our way through the infusion with "chemo humor." We laughed through the whole treatment. The lady next to us told the nurse she wanted whatever drug we were having. It was a memorable moment and again, God sent me angels. He always knew my limits and helped me at the time I needed it most.

Another week passed. When I arrived for my 11th Taxol treatment, I was very solemn. It was getting harder to stay focused and not look ahead. I had two more treatments and the torture would end. Some of the mental wall I had developed started to crumble. I thought about my mother through the whole treatment.

Tammy noticed I was more quiet than normal. We discussed my thoughts briefly. She reminded me that I was not my mother and that we had caught my breast cancer early. Both were true. Still, I felt bad.

Depression can easily overtake you when you are fighting cancer. The reality of being told you have cancer and the fight you need to barrel through treatments take a heavy toll on your psyche. Many patients take anxiety medicines to help counter the effects of the drugs on their emotions. I was one of the few that chose not to take any. I was concerned they would create more problems for me. In the past, I usually halved the dosage requirements of any type of medication because I reacted so strongly to a full dose. I personally think the chemotherapy drugs had the same effect. They too caused a strong reaction in me.

MARCH FORTH

As I finished my 11th Taxol treatment, I began to feel the letdown. I knew I could not take much more of this treatment. It was the first time I allowed that thought to enter my head. It was plain to see that the side effects were ravaging my body. I hurt. I was nauseated. My muscles were extremely weak, and it was taking all my energy to move or sit. I could hardly climb stairs any more without great pain. When I walked, I had foot drop. I could no longer pull my toes up with each step because my muscles were weak. I walked with a stomp. My feet were numb. I was light-headed most of the time. My belly was swollen and I looked like I was pregnant.

My nervous system was constantly making me shake. Most of my fingernails were dead. My skin was dry; none of my glands was producing oil. My eyes were dry. The walls of my nostrils were so damaged, I could not breathe through them anymore. My mouth was full of blisters as far as I could see down my throat. My tongue was swollen. I had acid reflux and my stomach hurt. My body hurt any place my comfy couch touched it. My brain was fried. I could not remember much except this pain. But I had to stay focused. Though I was extremely exhausted, I could not sleep because my body was so stressed. It could not rest. I was holding fluid and my blood pressure was rising. My body was totally out of sync.

I journeyed through my final week telling myself _one more!_ It was the only thing that kept me going. During the weekend before my final infusion, I went to an outdoor party. It was all I could do to sit through the festivities. I could no longer take the heat or the socializing. I went into the house and sat in a recliner and cried. I was scared to take the last treatment. I thought it would take me over the edge and kill me. I did not recover this last week at all.

On August 3, 2009, I went to the oncology office to receive my 12th and final Taxol treatment. During my office visit, I started explaining to the doctor how I felt. My voice started wavering and my eyes began to water. This was the first time I had broken down during any of my doctor visits.

After listening to my symptoms, the doctor cancelled my final Taxol treatment. He stated the additional benefit of the treatment would not outweigh the side effects it would give me. I started to cry, but stopped. The wall I had built over the past seven months shut down my emotions quickly. I wanted to cry, but the wall would not let me.

I came out of the doctor's office and saw Tammy. She greeted me with a hug and a gift. My eyes were watering. I wanted to let go of the wall, but I couldn't. My wall had been built strongly and securely. I found it would take several months after this ordeal to detoxify my spirit and mind and let my emotions flow. I continued to *March Forth!*

29

HEALING AND RECOVERY

The next several months, I focused on healing and re-covering from the chemotherapy side effects. Each day I improved physically and mentally. It was like going through puberty again. My whole body was growing and producing new cells. It took energy to heal and it was a slow, exhausting process.

I did not realize how physically and mentally ex-hausting the treatment had been for me until a month had passed. My focus on surviving each day had blinded me to what the drugs were actually doing to my body. Once my focus could turn to healing, the extreme tired-ness I felt turned into utter exhaustion.

I started sleeping soundly. I slept. Then, I slept, again. Whenever I would awaken, I would be in the same posi-tion as when I'd fallen asleep, whether I'd slept two hours or 10 hours. I did not move. My body was exhausted.

One time I fell asleep in an awkward position. I awoke the next day with a painful pinched nerve in my back. After that incident, I had to make a conscious effort to fall asleep in a proper position.

I saw several great changes in the month following

the last chemotherapy treatment. The nausea and burning in my stomach continued but gradually decreased. The blisters in my mouth and throat disappeared. My hair grew rapidly. I could no longer make suction sounds on my bare head with my hand. (Hey, I had to humor my boys somehow!) The skin on my arms and legs began to tingle. It felt like something was crawling under my skin. The numbness in my feet decreased; however, it never completely disappeared.

Although I was improving overall, some things did not improve. Chemo brain continued to affect my thinking. The aching, burning, and painful sensations I felt in my muscles and joints also increased.

Following the chemotherapy treatment, movement became a vicious circle. Standing and walking created pain, but continuous movement decreased the pain. Continuous movement created exhaustion. Exhaustion made me rest. Resting made my joints and muscles hurt. The exhaustion and tiredness would continue to affect my thinking.

My body hurt for several months following treatment. It hurt for someone or something to touch it. I struggled to lie in my bed at night because even my bed hurt my body. Shortly after completing my chemotherapy treatment, I went to the store and bought a memory foam mattress pad. I doubled it over and laid it on my side of the bed. The foam helped suspend my body's pressure points against the mattress. I slept mostly on my side to reduce the amount of contact points between my body and the bed. I slept with a pillow between my knees to prevent my knees from touching each other. This helped immensely to reduce the pain. (I continued to use the foam pad and pillow for over a year.) Sometimes the pain was too intense while I was lying in bed and pain would keep me awake. In the middle of the night, I would get up and recline on my comfy couch. The couch's softness would help alleviate the pain. Simply put—my body hurt.

Several months after my last chemotherapy treatment, the pain in my muscles and joints continued. The simple tasks of sitting, standing, walking, and climbing steps were painful. They were major events in my day. Sometimes when I would attempt to stand, I would collapse because of the pain. At times, it was too painful to move.

Getting out of bed each morning was the toughest. I would sit on the edge of my bed mentally preparing myself to stand and walk. I knew the task would make me hurt. I would stand and lean on my treadmill, gradually shifting my weight to my legs. Then I would begin to walk. The first 20 steps were the hardest. Again, the more activity I did, the easier it was to move. It was always toughest trying to move after a period of inactivity. Finally, in March 2010, I felt some relief from the pain. Eight months after my last chemotherapy treatment, my joints and muscles finally made a turn for the better.

As my physical side effects continued to heal, my mental side effects became more prominent. The reality of being treated for breast cancer weighed on my mind. I had been so busy trying to survive the treatment and surgery, and cope with the sudden decisions I had to make after my diagnosis that my mental exhaustion had begun to surpass my physical exhaustion. I now began to process what had happened to me.

Mentally, I was not progressing as fast as I thought I should be. I was still struggling with the chemo brain. It was still hard for me to transfer words from my brain to my mouth. My memory would come and go, especially when I was tired. The simplest of tasks exhausted me. Since I tired easily, my frustrations increased.

My sons' schedules kept me busy. I would rest all day so I could attend their events at night. When I arrived at these events, my energy would be rapidly depleted. I felt like a huge rechargeable battery. Once the battery ran down, I could not move or talk. I would have to rest at the event before I was able to move again. I had to re-charge the battery before I could even go home. If some-one came up to talk to me during this recharging phase, I did not have the energy to talk back. I might have forgot-ten her name even if I had just been talking to her. When my energy ran out, I was down for the count.

It was embarrassing. This was occurring as late as seven months after my last chemotherapy treatment. I became more secure if Steve or a friend was with me. They could help me get home or pick up the conversa-tion so I could recharge. Therefore, most times I did not leave home alone until I became stronger.

Some people assumed my side effects would immedi-ately go away after I completed my last treatment. This simply was not the case. Research shows healing may take as much as two to three years following chemotherapy treatment. I thought I would rebound quicker, but it was apparent I was not.

As the months passed, my mental perceptiveness was returning. However, it lagged behind the astuteness I'd had before chemotherapy. I still had lapses as well. It was frustrating. No matter how hard I wanted to assimilate back into my social circle, I was still struggling with my mental acuity. I started having doubts that it would ever return to the normal state I'd had before chemotherapy treatments.

Beginning in April 2010, I began evaluating my progress monthly. I could not see the daily improvements but did notice great strides on a monthly basis. Slowly but surely, I was improving. It felt good to see progress and improvements in my mental and physical well-being.

In May 2010, the school year was coming to an end. I was looking forward to summer vacation with Corey and Clay. I wanted to make up for the time with them that I had lost the previous summer while I was going through chemotherapy. However, summer vacation was more of a challenge for me than I expected.

Recovering from chemotherapy with two teenagers in the house was about as challenging as putting a thick rope through the eye of a sewing needle. It was a bigger challenge than I had anticipated. To say the least, it left me extremely nervous and exhausted.

The demands on my time and energy increased with my sons home for summer vacation. I would soon learn that their demands exhausted my battery quickly and efficiently. I still could not multitask like I had before I was diagnosed. Thus, it was a challenge to keep focused on attending to their needs.

I spent a lot of energy running to and from their events throughout the summer. However, it was their bickering with each other that got on my nerves the most. Trying to use logic with teenagers when they were arguing with each other was almost a bigger task than taking a chemotherapy treatment! I would lose my patience and begin yelling at them about the dumbest things. And losing my temper would send me into a tailspin mentally and leave me exhausted physically. I could exhaust my battery within minutes during one of these clashes. I immediately would have to lie down and rest.

I was disappointed in myself. I thought I had physically progressed more than I really had. I told Steve I felt like I had taken two steps backwards.

Somehow my kids and I survived the summer vacation. They returned to school in the fall. For the first time in my life, I looked forward to my kids going back to school. This _March Forth_ depressed me. I loved my kids, but I felt like I was a terrible mom. However, I knew with their return to school, I would make greater strides in returning to good health. I would continue to improve until I was faced with another surprise in October 2010.

30

NO HAIR TO BE FOUND

During chemotherapy, I lost all of my hair. Everywhere!
All of my eyelashes, eyebrows, nose hair, arm hair, leg
hair, and even pubic hair was gone. Nothing! I was bald
everywhere!

I had to make some adjustments after I lost my hair.
During the cold weather, I had no hair to provide insula-
tion for my head. My head and ears were cold. Therefore,
I slept with a sock hat on my head at night to keep warm.

During warmer weather, I would overheat. My hair
had provided shade from the direct sunlight and the
day's heat and humidity. I missed the natural cooling effect it had on my head. Since I had no hair, the sweat
evaporated quickly and I would overheat more rapidly.

However, I found some advantages of not having
hair. I didn't have to wake up in the morning and fix it. I
could massage my head easily. I didn't have to shampoo
daily. However, I did miss the smell and feel of my hair.
Some days I would shampoo my bald head.

Most times I wore a golf cap. If I was going to a special event, then I wore my wig. I loved telling people we
were late because I was fixing my hair, especially when

I was wearing only the golf cap. I also enjoyed asking people around me if I could borrow a hairbrush or comb.

Two months after I finished my Red Devil Cocktails, I had a pleasant surprise. Small white fuzz began to grow on my head. My hair was finally beginning to grow again!

I had heard lots of postchemotherapy hair stories. Some hair grew back in different colors and shades. Some hair grew back wavy or curly. It didn't matter to me. I just wanted *any* hair to grow back on my head. I hoped it would be a full head of hair and not patches, as some chemo patients experienced postchemotherapy.

As I watched my hair grow, it was a small light at the end of my recovery tunnel. Some people told me it was coming back blonde. Others told me it was coming back white. I didn't care if-they were color-blind or just being kind—I had hair growing on my head!

A month after chemotherapy, I had a breakthrough while walking one day. I could feel the wind blow through the few small strands of hair on my head. What a feeling! It felt like the angels were massaging my head. I could also detect a small scent of the oil that my hair was now producing. The scent lingered if I positioned my head a certain way when the wind blew. I had not realized this scent was gone until the wind blew through what little hair I had on my head that day. Wow! The little things in life we take for granted.

My hair was growing. By the end of October 2009, I went to my hairstylist to have the few uneven strands of hair that grew longer than the rest cut off. At that time, my hair was about an inch in length and very wavy. My hairstylist convinced me it was healthier for my hair to grow without the hat. Thus, I decided to stop wearing my golf cap.

Exposing my head without my golf cap was a big step. I was not comfortable at first. I kept the golf cap with me, readily available in case I could not handle going out in public. After a couple of weeks, it didn't matter whether I had the golf cap with me or not. I was accepting the battle I had recently completed. My hair was my badge of honor. I _was_ returning to "normal."

In late November 2009, I met Tammy for lunch. It was the first time we had seen each other in three months. She and I had recently completed our first postchemotherapy CT scans. The scans were our first checks to verify no cancer was present. Both our tests were negative. We were celebrating.

She also had stopped wearing her hair cover. We laughed when we saw each other for the first time. We both had buzz cuts. Then we laughed at the surrounding customers because they were staring at us. (You don't see two women with buzz cuts together often.)

Suddenly, I saw my former boss across the way. I walked over to talk to him. I said hello and asked him how he was doing. He looked at me and said, "Pardon me, your face looks familiar, Miss, but I don't know who you are." I hadn't meant to embarrass him, but I had. I introduced myself again and we had a good laugh. On the other hand, _I_ was not embarrassed. I had been through hell and was glad I was standing in a restaurant able to eat something. I forgot about the shock factor of my appearance for someone who had not gradually seen my physical changes as I progressed through my journey.

As my hair grew, the colors came back in stages. First the white/blonde color grew. Then gray, black, brown, and auburn colors arrived, in that order. I had a variety of colors. However, I did have two large gray patches of hair in places I had not had them before the chemotherapy treatments. This journey had certainly aged me.

As time passed, the curl in my hair tightened. Clay would tease me, telling me I had an Afro. He would place my pick comb in my hair. We laughed.

Eight months later, in June 2010, I went to my hairdresser for highlights. This was a milestone. My hair had grown enough that I could style it. My hairstylist was so excited to help me. The suspense grew as she removed the hair color application cap. Tears welled into my eyes. *Another milestone toward normality reached,* I thought. She remarked how thick and full my hair was, unlike that of most chemotherapy patients. I credited it to all the vitamin supplements, exercise, and healthy foods I continued to feed my body before, during, and after my treatment.

On her recommendation, I bought some scented hemp oil to help moisturize my hair. The chemotherapy had made my hair extremely dry. With the addition of the highlights, I needed the extra conditioning. Although my hairstylist recommended applying the hemp oil once or twice a day, my hair was so dry I applied it six or seven times a day. I also added a lightly scented body splash to add fragrance to my hair.

Wow! *What a difference a year made,* I thought. Last

year at this time, I could hardly sit up. Now, I was doing something as frivolous as applying highlights to my hair. **_March Forth_** to all of you who have lost your hair because of chemotherapy! It _will_ grow back!

31

ADVICE AND HELP FOR LOVED ONES AND PATIENTS

Although the treatments were exhausting for me, they were also extremely exhausting for my caregivers, especially Steve. I noticed the exhaustion on his face as he tried to keep the household running and also maintain his work schedule. His exhaustion was apparent the weeks following my last treatment. He would lie on the couch after supper and almost immediately fall into a deep sleep. He continued this for several weeks before he too could recover some of his stamina. He had amazing strength and energy throughout and following my treatment. His efforts were a true demonstration of his love for me, and I truly thank him from the bottom of my heart for being there for me.

After experiencing the diagnosis and treatment of and recovery from breast cancer, I gained a lot of insight into what it's like to be touched by breast cancer. I would like to share some of these experiences and my advice to others in the same position. The thoughts and ideas that follow are my perceptions of what people affected by cancer need.

- A lot of people diagnosed with cancer have positive outcomes. This is important for the patient, caregiver, and friends to remember. Stay positive and hopeful throughout the treatment. *This is the most important item to remember for anyone touched by cancer!*
- People diagnosed with cancer *do not* want to hear about others who have been diagnosed with cancer. They do not want to hear the details about another person's diagnosis. They especially do not want to hear the details of how badly the cancer has affected the other person. Definitely, *do not* tell them the other person is almost dead or has died from cancer. This is a common complaint I hear from other individuals and families who have been diagnosed with or affected by cancer. I have heard the most horrific stages and details of other people's cancer while I was going through treatment! This is the most insensitive and negative remark you can make to individuals recently diagnosed with or receiving treatment for cancer. It really defeats their efforts to fight their own battle. People diagnosed with cancer will ask if they want to hear more information. But in the meantime, *if the person diagnosed with the cancer doesn't ask, don't tell.*
- If a friend or family member has to visit:
  1. Make the visit short.

2. Visit at the end (not the beginning) of the treatment week.

3. Do not expect the patient to speak much.

4. During your visits, immediately wash your hands to prevent the spread of germs. The patient's immune system is compromised and visits can bring unwanted sickness.

5. Call before you come and ask if the patient is able to have visitors. Remember, the patient wants to visit, but some days that is impossible. <u>Note</u>: Different chemotherapies have different side effects. Some side effects are more severe or more manageable than others.

6. If the patient does not want visitors, call another day to arrange a visit. A patient receiving chemotherapy treatment needs contact with friends and family—but at certain times. When I was taking my Red Devil Cocktails, it was impossible to visit immediately following treatments. _Short_ visits toward the end of the treatment week worked best for me.

7. Do not insist on coming, even if only for a short visit (unless, of course, you are visiting other family members).

8. Please do not come to visit with pity in your eyes. This is negative energy. It will rob the patient of the positive energy needed to fight this battle. Convey confidence that your friend will survive and beat the disease. Here are some encouraging comments you might make: "I am

sorry you have to go through this, but know I am here for you." "I know you are going to do your best." "You are a strong person." "You are doing great." Remember, concentrate on the positives and dismiss the negatives.

9. If you can't visit, call and leave positive messages on the answering machine. If patients feel like talking, they can answer the phone. If they cannot talk, the positive voice and message will help brighten their day. They can listen to the message later perhaps when it is most needed. I loved phone calls but could not always talk. If someone did leave a message, I sometimes replayed it if I was at a critical point in my treatment. Positive words and encouragement did wonders for me when I was trying to survive, minute by minute and second by second.

- E-mail and text encouragement. Again, a patient going through treatment is able to read and reread these written encouragements. They also give the patient an opportunity to respond, later when the pain is more manageable.

- Refrain from saying "I know how you feel!" Chemotherapy affects each patient differently. There are some common side effects, but each individual responds differently. You do _not_ know how they feel!

- Asking "What can I do for you?" is good. Better yet, call and offer to _specifically_ bring something or _specifically_ do something. "I want to bring a casserole; what day can I bring it?" "I can mow the lawn; what day may I come?" "I can do the laundry; when can I come?" "I can pick up your child and bring him home." "I am at the grocery; can I bring you something?" When you present the specific options, it is harder for the patient to dismiss help. Patients may be too proud to ask for help when they really do need it. It also lightens their organizing load. Remember, they are already overwhelmed with treatments and issues surrounding the diagnosis and, due to the chemotherapy, probably not thinking clearly.

- Remember, chemotherapy causes chemo brain in a patient's brain, making it hard to think straight. Simple decisions are hard to make. Be supportive. If they forget something, help patients remember. Don't patronize them for forgetting.

- Organize a food schedule for the family who has been affected. Some families are more organized than others, but when the main organizer is the patient, meal planning becomes an additional burden for the family. I had a great friend, Valerie (an angel), organize this for Steve. We scheduled the food every other day. She then handed the schedule to our family members, who could easily make additions and corrections. (This worked great for us.)

- If you choose to bring food without making previous arrangements, make sure the food can be frozen and reheated later. Some other kind soul may have brought food on the same day you are bringing yours. The family may have too much food in one day. (Some days the family may not have any food, other days too much.)

- Don't second-guess the treatment decisions a patient has made. You are more than likely not as well informed about the person's diagnosis and second-guessing treatment decisions is not helpful. Each cancer diagnosis is different. Facts are important, and ignorance is not bliss in this situation.

- Encourage! Encourage! Encourage!

- Do not insinuate that a special food or supplement will stop cancer. Remember, everyone wants to fix this disease. No miracle food or drug has been found to cure cancer at this point in time or we all would be taking it.

- Offer the patient a ride to doctor appointments, infusions, the grocery store, or any other appointment. You can also pick up prescriptions, dry cleaning, and groceries or do yard work or house cleaning.

- Sit with a patient through an infusion or during the day, at home. However, don't expect the patient to talk.

- Send a positive or inspiring greeting card. Remember, it needs to be optimistic or comical and not gloomy. Sometimes I could not open my cards for several days following treatments because I was too sick or tired. However, knowing someone took the time and effort to send a card helps a patient throughout the process. It gives the patient a small, focused goal to open the card. Send a second card if the treatment takes several months. It makes patients feel they have not been forgotten.

- Transport the patient's children to and from their events, practices, and school. Remember, what may be the smallest gesture to you may be a huge undertaking for a chemotherapy patient. (Chemotherapy patients exhaust easily.)
- If you have no time to cook, buy a restaurant gift card. This will help the patient's family. Remember, chemotherapy patients want _bland,_ comforting food. Cold watermelon, slushies, and ice cream are also comforting.
- Do not tell the patient it was too upsetting or tough for you to call or visit. Think about that statement! You are telling the patient you have abandoned him or her. Trust me: The patient feels isolated already because of the diagnosis and at the mercy of the cancer treatment. Believe me, I know it is hard for others to accept a diagnosis about a friend or family member, but it is harder for the patient to accept the diagnosis. _You have a choice_ whether to accept or deal with a diagnosis. _I did not have a choice_. No patient has a choice when cancer happens. _I had to accept the diagnosis_ and then make logical decisions for treatment. If face-to-face contact is too hard for you, call or send a card. But to tell a patient it's too upsetting to visit and then not call or e-mail is a statement in itself. You have

abandoned this relationship and friendship.

- Do not avoid the patient. It is defeating. The patient is still the same person you loved and cared for before diagnosis. If you choose to avoid your friend or family member, you are telling the patient "when the chips are down, I'm not available. When you are healthy again, I'll be back." A patient needs your support at _all_ times, the good and the bad.

- Cancer tests friendships, relationships, and marriages. It percolates through the people in your life, from the top to the bottom. It clarifies what and who is important in your life. Sometimes our relationships are not what we thought they were before we were diagnosed. You will find out who truly is there to help you after this experience.

- All people feel helpless and scared when their friends or family members have been diagnosed with cancer. These are normal feelings, but _do not pull away from them._ Everyone can contribute to the situation by encouraging and staying positive. I felt helpless when Mom was diagnosed. I could not help her. It was her battle. However, as painful as it was to see her go through her diagnosis and treatments, I put my feelings aside and tried to be positive, happy, and optimistic when I was around her. This is what I could do to help. Some people internalize their fears and can't get past them. It is important to get past these fears and stay connected to the cancer patient. Remember, it is scary for your friends and family but extremely scary for the cancer patient.

- A patient diagnosed with cancer needs to focus on being positive. Maintain your humor. I watched the "*Golden Girls*" sitcom repeatedly. The show made me laugh.
- I suggest taking the following items with you during chemotherapy treatment:
    1. A small *bland snack*. (I packed an egg and cheese sandwich.)
    2. *Lemon drops*—they help with nausea and the taste of chemicals in the mouth during infusion.
    3. A *jacket* or *blanket*—infusion of the fluids tends to make you cold.
    4. *MP3 player* or *radio* for listening to soothing music.
    5. *Earplugs*—to keep your listening private. I was unable to read during the infusion because the drugs affected my brain and eyes. Others might be more successful with reading material.
    6. *Nausea medicine*, if it has been prescribed.
- Give the caretaker a break. Take them to a movie, a ballgame, or lunch. If the patient has children, invite them over for a play date. Remember, cancer affects everyone in the household.
- Following chemotherapy treatments, take a friend to the initial follow-up scans and tests and doctor visit for moral support. The first and second

scans and tests are the most emotionally challenging visits following chemotherapy. Your mind and body are still healing from the effects of chemotherapy. Anxiety levels are high and the mind can be swamped with questions: *Did the chemotherapy work? Are my scans going to be clear?* And so on.

Remember, the most important thing you can do for someone going through this crisis is to offer support, encouragement, and positive reinforcement.

32

RANDOM THOUGHTS

During my journey I had a few thoughts and experiences, some humorous, that I want to share with you.

"I Don't Know How You Did That"

Whenever I would explain to someone what I was experiencing through the peak of the churn and burn, he or she would respond, "I don't know how you did that" or "I don't think I could do that." I didn't have a choice. It was either lie down and never get back up or get through it. Just like any human being experiencing life-changing incidents or tragedies, I got through it. If life knocks you down, you get back up. Make an effort to help yourself. No matter how big or little the effort is, keep trying. You are successful as long as you never, ever give up.

Many times when I was at the peak of my churn and burn, I would remind myself that someone someplace somewhere was in a more difficult position or more pain than I was. I tried to make little of my pain. When I came to a position where I could not handle the pain, I walked and talked with God. I let Him carry me. I leaned on

Him for support until I could handle it myself. Again, He bridged my seconds together to help me until I could help myself again. Remember, God helps those who help themselves. Simply put, I would not have made it without my faith and do not know how others survive without it.

It's All about the Goal

Cancer treatment was all about goals. I finish this treatment by establishing long-term, short-term, and very short-term goals. In the beginning of the treatment, it was about survival. I successfully passed the pain by concentrating on seconds at a time. At the beginning of treatment, you need to have a plan, for managing your treatment by establishing attainable goals. Managing the small goals will help you achieve the bigger ones. Staying focused is the number one priority in achieving these goals.

"I'm Having a Bad Day"

I had a lady visit me shortly after one of my chemotherapy sessions. Although I was taking Taxol, which was less harsh than the Red Devil Cocktails, the cumulative effect of the drug was taking its toll on my mind and body.

"I'm having a bad day," she said.

"Why is that?" I asked.

She'd had a contractor deliver a product to her house. The contractor had brought the wrong product, damaged the driveway, and placed the product in the wrong area. I listened intently to her frustrations as she explained in good humor how her day had unfolded. In the process of listening to her "bad day" story, I couldn't help but let my thoughts wander. *I would be glad to switch places with her for the day*, I thought.

When she finished telling me about her day, I sat and looked at her. Smiling, I said, "Well, I am really sorry about your bad day. I can sympathize with you, but I am having a bad day, too. I would be more than glad to trade places with you if that would help." We both laughed.

The "bad day" lies in the eye of the beholder. One person's bad day can seem insignificant to others who are facing health and pain issues. Again, pain has a tendency to clarify what really is important. It amounts to a crash course on personal priorities. Remember, empathy runs both ways.

Mentally Processing the Diagnosis

Your mental state is put on overload when you are told you have cancer. First, you are in shock. Then, your mind goes numb. Next, your mind starts to race with all sorts of thoughts. *Am I going to die? What will happen to my kids? How much time do I have left? My God, I am only 49 years old! I'm healthy! How did this happen? I still have a lot of things I need to teach my kids!* I felt like I had been handed a death sentence. I worried about my family. A gamut of thoughts swirled in my head. At times I thought my head would explode! I could not physically control what had happened to me. I felt helpless. When this happens, focus on staying positive. Take deep breaths to reduce the anxiety.

Great Bedside Manner

In September 2009, I went for my first CT/PET scan post-chemotherapy. Thank goodness, my friend Erum insisted she take me to my appointment. This was my first check for cancer following chemotherapy treatment. I was nervous.

As we drove to the appointment, my anxiety began to rise. I had not prepared for this mental challenge. *What if none of the surgery, chemotherapy, and preventive medicine had worked? What if the scan showed more cancer? What if . . . ?* Erum knew I was experiencing these thoughts and was constantly grounding me telling me that things were going to be OK.

We waited in the lobby for my name, to be called. When the attendant announced my name, Erum and I both stood. She wished me good luck. The attendant told us there was a waiting room in the back near the scanning room for family members. I looked at Erum and she looked at me and we both laughed. I said, "Sure! She is family. Come on back, Erum!" She smiled and I smiled. I said, "In fact, we are sisters!" The male attendant laughed. I said, "In fact we are not only sisters, we are twins!" All of us were chuckling loudly then. You see, I have light hair, very fair skin, and blue eyes. Erum has dark olive skin, black hair, and dark brown eyes. The humor broke my anxiety.

Poor Bedside Manner

In November 2009, I went for my second CT/PET scan. It had been three months since I'd finished my chemotherapy. My name was called and I proceeded to a room to prep for my test. The employee set up an IV to administer the radioactive material into my arm and left. The only words she spoke were, "Do not move." Since I'd had this test three months earlier, I knew the procedure, but I was concerned about her poor bedside manner.

The radioactive infusion took approximately 45 minutes. I slept because I was still experiencing exhaustion. When it was time for my scan, she returned to take me to the scanning machine room. She told me to lie on the scanning bed. I stopped her. I informed her that I was wearing my prosthesis and would need to remove it for the scan. (For the previous test, a male employee had discretely helped me with this process.) She told me to "Just pull it out!" I told her I was not going to just pull it out! "Please give me a hospital gown," I requested. She stood there and waited for me to change. I requested a room so I could change into the hospital gown in privacy. I was ticked.

When I finished my scan, she returned and picked up my bra, which contained the prosthesis. She looked over the bra, turned it over, and looked at the other side of the bra! She then pulled the prosthesis out of the support bra, felt it, and looked it over as well! She then handed the separate pieces back to me. I was completely offended and felt violated. This prosthesis was a part of me.

Would a person manipulate a saline breast inserted in a woman's body? If she would have asked, I would have shown her. I was proud of my prosthesis. I requested that I not to have her in the future. She was a nightmare.

What a Difference a Year Makes

In July 2010, I was bringing my children home from the 4-H Fair. I was very tired. My joints continued to hurt but were feeling better than during the previous months. My legs were still weak. The smallest of efforts exhausted me. It was dark as I was driving home. I was talking to my kids and became distracted and missed the turn onto the road to go home. I briefly became confused about where I was and questioned whether or not I had indeed missed my road. The chemo brain reared its ugly head once again. The exhaustion and tiredness that hit me suddenly caused my confusion. For a few seconds, I was anxious, but my mind quickly got its bearings. We made it home.

Though I was still struggling, I was nowhere near the depleted physical condition I'd had been at the 4-H Fair a year earlier. Then, the 4-H Fair had opened right after one of my chemotherapy treatments. I wanted to go to the fair and see Corey and Clay's 4-H projects, but it was not likely to happen since I had completed my chemo treatment that afternoon. After my treatment, I went home and sat on my comfy couch. My kids and Steve went to play a flag football game. As I sat on the couch, I thought how badly I wanted to see the kids' 4-H projects. When they returned from the game, I decided I would try very hard to make it to the fair that evening. I borrowed my dad's wheeled walker with a basket and seat on it, packed a bottle of water, and went to the fair. Clay pushed me around on the rolling walker so I could see the projects.

As Clay pushed the walker, I grabbed the water bottle I had placed in the basket and found it empty. I had accidentally forgotten to tighten the lid, and there was a trail of water throughout the project display building. We laughed as we saw that the trail led to my walker. We refilled my bottle and continued. We stopped to talk to someone I knew and my nose began to bleed. I had to scramble for a Kleenex. After I saw my sons' projects, we started home. I ran into a friend as we left. She stopped and talked to me and I could not remember her name and I had to apologize for forgetting. We finally made it home. I was in pain. The trip had almost been too much for me.

What a Difference a Month Makes

In August 2010, Clay and I went to my friend's house to swim. At least I was going to _try_ to swim. We were in the pool almost two hours. I sat on a float most of the time, maintaining my balance in the water. I made a comment that a month ago I would not have been able to hold myself up on the float. When I drove home, it was after 10:00 p.m. It was the first time in a long time I had driven that late at night.

When I got home, I immediately went to bed and slept soundly through the night. My phone's alarm awakened me the next morning. When I woke up, I realized I had been dreaming. It was the first time I could recall having a dream since I'd started chemotherapy.

Corey's Confirmation

In March 2010, I attended Corey's confirmation at our church. It was one of those rare milestones in a child's life that a parent wants to experience. It was emotional for me to see him make his commitment. I felt I could not do anything more important for him in his life than to help him come to know God. We had been taking the boys to church since they were born. It was a part of our life. Seeing him make this commitment, statement of faith, and belief in the Trinity gave me the comfort that no matter what happens today, tomorrow, or EVER, Corey's relationship with and faith in God would be there! It was another thing to cross off my "bucket list."

33

TWO STEPS FORWARD AND ONE STEP BACK

In mid September 2010, I was having an intermittent, sharp pain in my right breast. I'd had this pain before, but for some reason the intensity had stepped up several notches. (During that week, we'd had high pressure, a full moon, and an equinox. Mother Nature often lets me know about my aches and pains!) I called my doctor and expressed my concerns. I was scheduled for an MRI.

The MRI found an object deep inside my breast but not in the location where I was having the sharp pain. My doctor advised me to have it biopsied. With my past history, I needed to eliminate any suspicious area.

The day following my biopsy, I was notified of my results. Nothing suspicious was found in the area where I was experiencing pain, just a benign fibroadenoma (harmless tumor). However, they found some atypical lobular hyperplasia cells (ALHC), which is an overgrowth of cells that do not appear normal, behind the fibroadenoma. I consulted with my oncologist and surgeon for my next move. I was advised to have the atypical cells removed.

The surgeon informed me that ALHC were not considered cancerous or precancerous cells. ALHC can appear and disappear at any time in a women's breast. However, research has shown that ALHC can also turn into cancer approximately 10 to 15 years later. Since they had found ALHC in my right breast and I had a previous history of lobular breast cancer, I had to be more aggressive with my treatment. Taking the advice of my doctors, I elected to remove my right breast. I scheduled myself for a prophylactic (risk-reducing) mastectomy.

I was disappointed and angry. I had hoped a cure would have been found before I had to face another mastectomy. I had hoped to be diagnosed free of any type of atypical, precancerous, or cancerous cells until research provided a cure. I'd fallen short of this goal, and I felt defeated. I'd lost a new battle in an ongoing war.

Although I felt I had taken a step backwards, I forced myself to focus on the positive. I was still cancer free. *I was still winning the war.* By removing my right breast, I would reduce my breast cancer risk significantly. No lymph nodes would be removed this time, so my lymphatic system would not be compromised. Since no lymph nodes were being removed, I would not have the pain or the loss of sensation under my arm that I'd had with the previous mastectomy. No chemotherapy was needed. But, still, it was disheartening.

After making my decision to remove the breast, I contacted the surgeon to schedule my elective mastectomy. It was scheduled the following week as *outpatient surgery!*

I could not believe what I was hearing.

"Did you say outpatient surgery?!" I asked the nurse.

"Yes," she said.

Wow! I thought. I asked again just to be sure. I could not believe how much our health care is driven by what's best for the insurance companies. This was crazy! I went home to digest the fact that I was having a mastectomy *as an outpatient!* I christened it the "Drive-by Whack-a-Boob II" surgery. In fact, someone asked me where I was having the surgery and I replied, "McDonalds drive-thru!"

After digesting the fact that my surgery would be on an outpatient basis, I still felt fortunate. I had a facility and wonderful doctors who felt confident enough to perform this procedure in this manner. After all, the way the health insurance was going, I felt I might not be eligible for this type of surgery in the near future—maybe the government or my insurance company would dictate that this surgery was not necessary. (With all the changes happening in health care, I could face that possibility!) At least the government and insurance were not handing out take-home bags with "do-it-yourself kits" for mastectomies. At least not yet!

I kept myself busy the week preceding my surgery. I bought myself some roses and set them on the table. (It was another experience of death for me. I was going to lose my breast.) I was angry. I don't recall experiencing these thoughts concerning my initial mastectomy because I knew it was going to save my life. However, this time, anger enveloped me as I thought about losing my remaining breast.

Finally, on November 1, 2010, my surgery day arrived. I cried. I cried when I awoke. I cried all the way to the surgery center. I cried during admittance. I cried until I was given anesthesia. It was a big loss for me. After I awoke from the anesthesia, I just could not look down at my chest. I could not bear to see my flat chest.

In recovery, the nurses pushed the pain medicines. I received five doses of pain medicine from three different prescriptions. I was sent home four hours later and advised to take two more different prescriptions for pain. I was bombed.

For the next three days, I tried the prescription pain medicine, but it was not working for me. I called the surgical nurse and requested something different. She advised me to see another doctor for my pain. I called another doctor and I was given anxiety medicine. It did not take my pain away but it did make me rest, which was helpful. I felt the drive-by outpatient surgery for my mastectomy was not in my best interest. I highly recommend that anyone contemplating a mastectomy try to spend the night after in the hospital. After my mastectomy, I found out that I could have spent the night at the hospital if I had pushed the issue. Again, this was dictated by insurance policies.

The following two weeks postsurgery, I dealt with the physical side effects. I felt the pain of the surgical site, the inflamed lungs caused by a reaction to the anesthesia, and the physical shock to my nervous system from losing a body part. I was also dealing with the mental loss of losing both of my breasts. I was experiencing depression.

Once again, many of my angels arrived. Sara called to tell me "to mourn my loss," "the loss will make me stronger," and "many people still love you because you're the same person inside." Carol, Carolyn, Tammy, and others transported my sons and brought food; Penny sent several positive messages; Jim and Janet did kind deeds; Diana was with me in spirit from Texas, and so on. Again, these nice words and deeds, calls, e-mails and texts helped me greatly.

Losing a breast is mentally tough for any woman. When I lost the first breast, it was challenging. However, losing both breasts was indescrible.

I remember when my mother experienced her first mastectomy. Her attitude never changed. She was still positive, happy, and excited that she had rid herself of the breast that had cancer. (This is a lot like I felt, too.) She was upbeat when she came out of the surgery. I remember the nurses making comments about her positive attitude.

Six months later, she was experiencing some other issues with her healthy breast. Mom knew something was wrong. Thanks to her persistence, the surgeon ordered a biopsy. The biopsy was positive. She immediately needed another mastectomy. I remember Mom was different after the second mastectomy. It was as if some of the fire and drive behind her eyes was replaced with a question mark. She never talked to me about her thoughts, nor did I ask her about them. I could only guess what some of her thoughts were.

Now, I understand the question mark I saw behind

my mom's eyes. I cannot explain these feelings to others. They would not understand. But, I now know. Although my mom has passed, she continues to help me understand this process. I am not alone.

Using hindsight, I realized that last year I had leaned on the fact that I still had my right breast. But now I had none. Although I knew I would survive this loss, it was harder mentally to lose the second breast. I now realized I had not mourned my first lost breast because I had been intensely focused on surviving the chemotherapy treatment. (Again, pain has a way of bringing clarity and priority to your life.)

My second mastectomy allowed me to mourn my second lost breast as well as the first. The second mastectomy allowed feelings to surface that I had buried a year earlier. The more I talked to breast cancer survivors, I found each of us mourns at different times and different places. Some will mourn immediately after diagnosis. Some will mourn later, after they feel in control of themselves. In the meantime, we stay strong for the battle, never knowing if we will win the war.

Some of us will never mourn because we want to maintain our strength. We are all strong, and we are all survivors. However, during the process, I think we need to mourn to build our strength. The second mastectomy allowed me to finally mourn, which in turn allowed me to build my strength. This will be a continuous process for the rest of my life. It does get easier as time passes.

I suffered depression after my second mastectomy. Part of my depression was fueled by the insensitivity and ignorance of the insurance industry. How horrific is it for a woman to lose her breast and then fight the insurance process for prostheses?! It made my second mastectomy an exhausting nightmare. It was inexcusable. I dealt with the insurance company for several hours almost every day for *three months* following surgery. The mental anguish was extremely hard while trying to physically recover from my mastectomy. I was mentally breaking down each time I contacted the insurance company. I filed an appeal with the insurance company based on the grounds of discrimination. I am awaiting the results of the appeal.

You can never fully understand how a person feels unless you have experienced a similar loss yourself—a miscarriage, or a loss of a husband, wife, or child. Nor can you really understand what someone feels about a cancer diagnosis or mastectomy. I think it is easy for someone who has not been diagnosed with breast cancer to state, "I would remove both breasts if it were me." But the decision to remove one's breasts is more complex than a glib opinion. Breasts are considered the feminine symbols of a woman. They contribute to a women's sex appeal. Sure, removing your breasts physically removes the cancer, but it does not address the emotional loss of losing both breasts. A part of me died. It is gone. Never will it be back. Reconstruction cannot bring it back either. It is important to grieve this loss. If reconstruction helps in any way, a woman should do it. Again, it is a personal choice.

Some of my friends had advised me to have a double

mastectomy the previous year. But I chose to do a unilateral mastectomy instead. I was confident in that decision. I based that decision on research and advice from my doctors. It was the right decision for me. As I said before, each woman's diagnosis is unique. Until you are in that position, you cannot know what it is like to make that decision.

I like the adage "Time heals all wounds." I do find through time I learn to balance my physical losses with spiritual gains. It is a process of mourning, increasing your mental and physical strength, and healing. It all takes time. Give yourself time and you will heal. I cannot rush the process but it is getting better. Time marches forth and I will *__March Forth__* as well. I can do all things through Christ which strengtheneth me (Philippians 4:13 KJV).

Another Coincidence!?

A couple of weeks after my second mastectomy, I realized another coincidence had occurred in my life. Another incident in my life had come full circle. Thirty years earlier, on November 1, 1980 (same date as my second mastectomy), when I was 20 twenty years old, I was in a wreck with a friend. The car was totaled. However, I walked away from the wreck with only a few pulled muscles and bruises because I was wearing my seat belt.

It was my friend's new car and my first ride in it. (I could not find the seat belt in the new car.) As we drove away, my friend stated, "Put your seat belt on!" We laughed, searched for the seat belts, and buckled them while driving down the road. Twenty minutes later, we were in the wreck.

The previous summer, I had been home from college, helping my friend's mother (an angel) with an odd job. She would pick me up and we would go to work in her car. Every time I entered the car, she said, "Put your seat belt on!" It became a habit after her insistence.

Had I not had my seat belt on the night of the wreck, I would have been ejected from the car. When we were hit, the car spun several times. While we were spinning, I was hanging out of the passenger door, looking at the pavement. I remember trying my hardest to stay in the car. If it were not for the seat belt, I shudder to think what could have happened to me in those few seconds.

The wreck had been a wake-up call for me in 1980. I was experiencing the growing pains one feels at that age. It gave me a second chance. It helped me refocus on what I needed to do with my life. The second mastectomy was another growing experience. It will help me refocus on what I need to do with my life again. For now, I will continue to _**March Forth!**_

34
A NEW YEAR

January 2011 was the beginning of a new year and arrived before I could blink. It had been a wearisome two months since my second mastectomy in November. My mental and physical energy had been taxed. I had not had as much downtime to heal from my surgery as I would have liked. Shortly after my mastectomy, my father's health declined, and Dad was admitted to the hospital. We eventually moved him in to an assisted living facility. While the family was trying to get Dad settled, the holidays were upon us. However, our holidays were overshadowed by a sudden death in the family. It seemed like one thing after another was happening. I told Steve, "God must have kept me busy so I would not have to think about my mastectomy." I was physically and mentally tired.

January 2011 also marked the two-year anniversary of when I had been initially diagnosed with breast cancer. It was hard to believe two years had come and gone. My struggle during this time to achieve and return to good health felt extremely longer. However, my strength and stamina were better each passing day on this road to recovery. I _was_ slowly and surely making strides to heal physically and mentally.

In March 2011, my family took a vacation. We went to the beach for Spring Break. The weather was perfect. I felt fortunate our family was able to make the trip. It was a much-needed break. I bought two new bathing suits especially fitted for my prostheses. The swimsuits were beautiful and held my prostheses perfectly. I could walk or swim on the beach without feeling self-conscious about my appearance.

As I sat on the beach, I realized how far I had progressed physically from this time a year earlier. I _was_ improving! However, I was still not as strong as I'd been before this whole journey had begun. On this trip, I was more energetic but still had to stop and rest while Steve and the boys ventured out. I would take a break and wait for them to come back to get me. After five glorious days on the beach, we drove the 10 hours back home. The break was something we all deserved more than I realized.

Emotionally, I was better than I'd been a year ago as well. I did not have the big emotional swings that I'd experienced throughout the previous year. I was contented and rested. As I was driving home, I realized I had finally put a lot of the two-year journey behind me. The trip to the beach had been good for all of us.

As we crossed the last stretch of the interstate towards home, we passed the building where I'd received my chemotherapy. The image immediately invoked a memory of the pain I had journeyed through. I started crying. I was not prepared for this emotional reaction. (This reminder of where I had been caused a crack in my wall, releasing some feelings so I could continue to heal.) I cried a few minutes and then quickly refocused on the positive, our vacation. I *Marched Forth* to what lay ahead of me. Home was waiting and so was our dog. She would be happy to see us. Again, I reminded myself how I had taken giant steps forward.

My journey continues. I progress and live each passing day with appreciation. Each day I am glad to rise in the morning to face the day and each night I am glad to go to bed because I am very tired. My health plan continues with preventive measures to prevent any cancer.

I take a prescribed aromatase inhibitor medicine daily. I will take this medicine for five years. Though it has side effects, it prevents my body from producing estrogen, which fed my breast cancer.

I take a prescribed bone-building medicine once a month to counter the negative effects of the aromatase inhibitor. (A lower estrogen level leads to a loss of bone density, which causes osteoporosis.) The bone-building medicine will prevent bone loss. However, it like the aromatase inhibitor also has its side effects.

I continue to schedule quarterly visits with my oncologist. These checks include the CBC test and CT/PET scans as needed to check for breast cancer reoccurrence.

I continue to adjust to my body's changes caused by these medicines and the loss of estrogen. I continue to strengthen my mental capacities and downplay the effects of the breast cancer in my life. I am constantly refocusing on *marching forward*.

Although I would not wish a cancer diagnosis on my worst enemy, I am a better person because of my experiences during this journey. I have concluded there are reasons why I had to experience this journey. But, no matter what they may be, I know I am an optimist and a survivor. No person can destroy or take those positive thoughts from me unless I let it happen. Therefore, I continue my journey for better health and healing.

As time *Marches Forth*, my anger decreases. I continue to work on my patience. I *am* getting mentally and physically stronger each day past the surgeries and chemotherapy treatments. I focus on remaining optimistic, hopeful, and happy. I try to inhale the good and exhale the bad. I attempt to surround myself with positive people and things. I try to encourage those who are not. Most times I am good at this. Sometimes I am not. My journey is to a great extent like a song I listened to during my chemotherapy treatments: "Don't Worry, Be Happy" by Bobby McFerrin.

Each day I survive, more solutions and better treatments become available for treating all cancers. This will benefit me and you. As I write this, I read that scientists have found that blocking a certain gene in our bodies prevents the breakdown of a certain protein. If this protein is protected, it will prevent cancer cells from spreading. I truly believe we are winning the war against cancer. In the meantime, I will continue to *March Forth* positively and stay hopeful that a cure will be found soon to protect me, my family, and your family.

Thus, I would like to finish sharing this two-year journey with you by paraphrasing one of my favorite Gladys Knight and the Pips songs: I have written a part of my life's story. I have had my share of life's ups and downs. Sometimes they were good times and sometimes they were bad times. But overall, fate has been kind to me. Whether the experiences were good or bad, I have made it through. God, my family, my extended family, my friends, and even strangers have been there for me between each line of the pain and glory. I am lucky to experience all of these times with these individuals because they helped me be who I am. I would like to tell each and every one of you a big "thank you" for being there for me. But most of all, I want to tell Steve, Lindsay, Corey, and Clay: "You're the Best Thing That Ever Happened to Me." I'm proud of you and love you all. ***March Forth!***

APPENDIX A
E-MAIL

I did not realize how many people I would reach when I began sending e-mail updates to friends and family. I sent e-mails containing information about my condition and experiences throughout my treatments. I think I learned as much about the people I sent the information to as they learned about me and how cancer treatments physically affect cancer patients. Many replied to tell me that the e-mails were very informative, educational, and inspirational. I even had some individuals who worked in the medical field tell me they had no clue what a chemo patient went through during chemotherapy treatments until they read my e-mails. The e-mails helped them become more sensitive to their patients and better caregivers.

Although my intention was to eliminate some exhausting groundwork of keeping everyone up to date, I had accidentally found a way to be helpful to others during a time that I needed _their_ help. I needed to send the e-mails to unload my thoughts and ground myself, but I also needed the responses to keep myself going day after day. At times, my cancer treatment brought me to my knees. When I was at my weakest point in the treatment cycle, I could go to my e-mail and find an inspirational message from someone or write. Thank you to each and every one of you who responded to me. It was a bigger help than you will ever realize.

When friends and families responded to my updates, it would energize me throughout my day. I had e-mail recipients forwarding the e-mails to other individuals. Word was reaching out to many people all over the United States, some of whom I didn't even know. As a result, people all over the country were putting me on their prayer lists. Some people sent the e-mails to other individuals who were also going through cancer treatments or had recently been diagnosed. I had a lady tell me she looked forward to my e-mails. She was receiving them from her sister-in-law, who was a friend of mine. She told me I was an inspiration to her and she wasn't sure if she could actually get through chemo if she ever had to go through it. This really touched me. These types of remarks would always increase my strength to tackle another portion of my day. I looked at her with admiration and said, "God can give you strength to get through anything." I knew she had been through the fire as well. She had lost her daughter, son-in-law, and two grandchildren in a tornado a few years earlier. We often look at others to give us inspiration and strength, but we rarely give ourselves credit for surviving some of the rougher times we have had to face in our own lives. The longer we live, the more things we all survive.

Thus, writing and e-mailing my updates served several purposes.

- I didn't have to keep repeating my status every time someone would ask or call. (You just don't have the strength or energy to talk when going through chemotherapy.)
- It gave Steve more time to handle the extra duties of being a caregiver, since he didn't have to repeat updates as well.
- By receiving updates via e-mail, my friends could keep up with me and I could better explain what was happening to me as I went through the process and treatments.
- It was my therapy. I wanted to communicate to my friends and family, but it was so tiring to talk. It actually hurt to talk. E-mailing allowed me to express my thoughts and share what I was internalizing, which helped combat my feelings of isolation and depression.
- It also allowed the recipients to respond. This is great mental support for those going through chemotherapy and allows friends and family to fulfill their need to help. Just a simple "hang in there" stuck with me the rest of the day.

What follows are some of my favorite e-mails chronicling my journey throughout diagnosis, treatment, and recovery. Some were written when the chemo drugs were hitting me full strength; therefore, some sentences may not entirely make sense. Again, I want to thank all of you responders and listeners.

God bless you all! And as always, ***March Forth!***

----- *Original Message* -----
From: Marci Schmitt
To: Undisclosed Recipients:
Sent: Monday, January 12, 2009
Subject: Mammogram and Biopsy results

January 12, 2009
I apologize for making this email seem so impersonal, but I have had several people request I call them about my results. I felt I could get the info out quicker at this pace. Thank you for all your thoughts and prayers.

As some of you may know, I had my annual mammogram completed last Tuesday. Again, the mammogram had some questionable spots and an ultrasound was completed on both breasts. During the ultrasound they found two questionable spots in the left breast and one in the right breast. A biopsy was scheduled a week later but moved up to last Thursday. Their suspicions were correct. The right breast is benign (which they thought all along but did as a precaution). The left breast has two spots that are irregular. It did come back as cancerous - Infiltrating Lobular Cancer. I am now in the process of scheduling another MRI and then talk to the surgeon about my options - lumpectomy, mastectomy radiation chemo etc. I will

take this one day at a time. I ask that you do think but not worry about me and keep your thoughts and prayers with me and others who are also facing a personal crisis. Again, thank you all for your thoughts and prayers. Thanks for your support.
Marci

----- Original Message -----
From: Marci Schmitt
To: Undisclosed Recipients:
Sent: Thursday, January 22, 2009
Subject: Progression of Breast Cancer

As some of you may know, I had questionable results on my Mammogram (Jan 6) which led to an MRI and 2 biopsies. In the last two weeks they confirmed I have Infiltrating Lobular Cancer in my left breast. Today Steve and I went to see the surgeon to hear all of the results and determine our next action. The right breast is benign but the left breast has two tumors - one five millimeters and one six millimeters. The MRI confirmed this and no more areas were diagnosed. Monday, I am going to have a bone scan to determine the pain in my ribs located below the tumor. The doctor did not believe this area is affected but is testing it to calm my fears. (Enough said there.) The doctor believes we have caught this at a very early stage and does not feel it has spread to the lymph nodes but this can only be determined when surgery is completed. They will test the lymph nodes during the surgery to see if the cancer has spread. Since breast cancer runs on my Mom's side of the family and given the fact she passed with breast cancer four years ago, I am having the breast cancer gene test completed. This is a fairly new test for breast cancer and just began testing locally in 2007. In fact when the lady had drawn my lab sample today, it was the first one she had done. Anyway, this will determine which method of surgery we decide.

If I test positive for the breast cancer gene, the writing is on the wall. I will have a bilateral mastectomy. I have no other choice.

If the test comes back negative, I will have a lumpectomy and radiation treatments in my left breast.

The gene test will take approximately 2-6 weeks before I get the results back. It is a very expensive test and insurance doesn't usually want to pay for it but it will determine the best option for me. The doctor said the cancer will not grow that fast and not to worry. (Easy for him to say!)

Anyway, the last two weeks have been like a whirlwind. It was as if someone punched me in the gut and took my breath away. It has been an anxious time. I will get through this and Steve will be a big help. It is just another chapter in my book of life and God is walking with me.

I really appreciate all the calls, emails, thoughts, prayers, cards etc. It has helped my spirit immensely. Thank you all for your concern and prayers.

And the big mug of margarita at Hacienda I had for lunch today, was extremely helpful as well (smile).

Thanks again for all the support and prayers. Please remember others who also may be facing their personal crisis as well.
Marci

----- Original Message -----
From: Marci Schmitt
To: Undisclosed Recipients:
Sent: Tuesday, February 03, 2009
Subject: February 3, 2009 Update:

Well I have had another interesting and very long week. Last Monday (Jan 26th) I had my bone scan. I had good news - it was clear. I am still waiting on the results of my breast cancer gene test. It now has been two weeks. (If you remember it takes 2-6 weeks to get the results and if the results are positive, I will be having bilateral surgery.)

Today (Feb 2), I went to the oncologist. He stated the same thing. If I test positive for the gene, I should have bilateral breast surgery and also I should have my ovaries removed. Since my cancer is estrogen fed, we need to stop my body from producing estrogen. (Starve the cancer and let the tumor die or be controlled basically.)

He has scheduled a MRI for my brain (could save some money there - they won't find anything) and a CT scan for my chest and abdominal cavity to make sure it has not spread. I will be having that Wednesday (Feb 4). He does not think the cancer is in this area but is taking the precautions through testing. He too felt the cancer was confined to a small area and the outlook good. I have already decided that I will completely remove the left breast with the tumors. I am not going to take any chances. He stated there would be a good chance I would not have to have radiation if I did that. We won't know until we check the lymph nodes during surgery. My next big decision will be to decide whether to have reconstruction or prosthesis.

I will begin taking ------to send my body into menopause. This will block the estrogen feeding the tumor hopefully. (Steve has been forewarned of upcoming behavior. This could be my revenge back to my kids. Hmmmmm! Teenagers and menopause!) Dr. ------stated this will give us time before surgery to see if this drug will work in my body. We are getting a head start.

The day ended on a bright note. I was at the checkout/registration table. The lady was trying to set up my appointments and was talking on the phone to someone. She stated her daughter was here to make the necessary appointments and she was looking at me. It finally registered and I asked if she was talking to me and she said yes! She thought I was the daughter and I finally told her I was the patient! We had a good laugh and of course I told her that she made my day. But then her next question was about my weight and then I became humbled again.

Thanks again for all the positive responses and prayers I have been receiving. They help me in more ways than I can express. Marci

----- *Original Message* -----
From: Marci Schmitt
To: Undisclosed Recipients:
Sent: Friday, February 20, 2009
Subject: results and surgery has been scheduled

Greetings,
Good news! My genetic test came back negative. This means I do not carry this particular gene for breast and ovarian cancer. (The BRCA test is a test . . . that has isolated a breast cancer gene in our body. If the gene is mutated, it produces breast and ovarian cancer. Since my health and family record fit the predetermined factors for taking this test, I elected to see if I was positive to help me make my decision on what surgery was needed.) Even though I was negative, we still have many other genes in our bodies that may cause cancer and have not been found by research. Thus, even though I was negative on the BRCA test, my doctor still believes it may very well be genetic because of my family history but we just don't know. However, because of this negative result, I will not be doing a double mastectomy or removing my ovaries at this time. My MRI and CT scan did not show any cancer which is great news as well. . . .

Anyway, my surgery is scheduled for March 4th which is "Action Day". (It is the only action day we have in our calendar year! Like a soldier - march forth-get it?) I will be having a unilateral mastectomy. Treatment following surgery will be one of the following: six months of chemo, three months of chemo, or none depending on the size of the tumor and/or lymph node involvement. (I am beginning to think the doctors are stretching this out so it becomes involved in the lymph nodes and then we can spend more money helping the drug companies!) I should be in the hospital one night (depending on the lymph nodes dissection) and recovery takes about 2-4 weeks. Chemo would start three weeks after surgery if it is needed. My oncologist stated that the ------ that I am now taking could reverse the progression of the cancer I now have. Since I will be on it exactly four weeks at my surgery date, he is anxious to see how my pathology report comes out. That would be a big plus for me if the ------works that well.

I decided to just do a unilateral mastectomy after researching, reading and listening to my doctors and nurses. Everyone has an opinion but until they walk in their own shoes with this life threatening/changing illness, the decision has to be what's right for that person. My chances of the cancer going to my right breast are now about 1 in 6 whereas before it was 1 in 8. We will be watching me like a hawk and technology will improve with time. Mainly, I did not want to live my life in fear and could not reasonably accept taking a part of me that was healthy unless it was dictated by tests or the doctors. Besides, if cancer is going to return, let's give it a target that I can find! Some say they would not want to worry about it with the checks etc. but let's face it - I have cancer and will be fighting its return the rest of my life.

Anyway, thanks again for the support and prayers I am receiving from you all. It has been one big spin after another and your support does help. Many of you have express helping me in some way especially after the surgery. Please email or call

------ *if you wish to help. She will be coordinating things so Steve and I can concentrate on post surgery recovery.*

Love and prayers for all of you.
Marci

----- *Original Message* -----
From: Marci Schmitt
To: Undisclosed Recipients:
Sent: Friday, March 06, 2009
Subject: surgery went well

Just a quick note. Surgery went well. No lymph node involvement. Considered Stage 1 and 95% cancer free. Treatment will be determined next week. Am home enjoying my meds.
Marci

----- *Original Message* -----
From: Marci Schmitt
To: Undisclosed Recipients:
Sent: Monday, March 9, 2009
Subject: Path report shows more cancer

Went to the oncologist today. On further review of the lymph nodes, one of the three did have a small tumor in the lymph node. . . . Now considered stage II cancer. Will now have full blown 6 months of chemo treatment which begins in two weeks. Will lose hair shortly after treatment and hopefully all cancer cells when treatment completed.
Marci

MARCH FORTH

----- *Original Message* -----
From: Marci Schmitt
To: Undisclosed Recipients:
Sent: Tuesday, March 17, 2009 12:05 PM
Subject: Update Mar 17

Happy St. Patrick's Day to all you Irish. Just found out I should be wearing orange (since I am Protestant) and not green (since I am not Catholic) today per the newspaper.

Anyway, I will be getting the rest of my staples taken out tomorrow. I also have been scheduled for same day surgery to put a port in my chest so all medicines and blood samples can be given easier. I was getting upset when I thought they were going to schedule it during my Purdue basketball game on Thursday.

I am getting my wig tomorrow or Thursday.

Physically, I am recovering a little bit each day from the mastectomy but not fast enough to satisfy me. I am still in pain somewhat and it makes me nauseous. I am down to two pain pills a day.

Emotionally, I cry once in awhile and then feel better a few days.

Spiritually, God is walking with me and holding my hand because I asked him to.

Monday, March 23 is my first dose of chemo.

Have a good spring break.
Marci

----- Original Message -----
From: Marci Schmitt
To: Undisclosed Recipients:
Sent: Tuesday, March 31, 2009
Subject: Update Mar 31

Hope everyone had a nice spring break. I've had better but kept telling myself things could be worse.

Well today is my 7th day after my first chemo treatment. I feel 100% better than last week. Each day I can see some difference in some positive progression from surgery. I still have pain in my arm and armpit. It feels like baler twine wrapped as tight as it can around that area. It was really doing a number on my nerves this weekend as I tried to take myself off the pain medicine. The pain medicine was not helping and the pain appears to be more (?) nerve.

It is very hard to read or write very long due to the side effects of the chemo and nausea medicine. It gives me a severe headache and my vision is blurry. It is hard to concentrate.

I continue to drink lots of water to flush my bladder. I have to drink three quarts a day to keep lesions from forming in my bladder.

My feet did go numb last week but have come back somewhat

this week. Then because I was drinking so much water my feet were cramping. My doctor did put me on additional vitamins to counter some of these side effects. However, I am craving salt and protein and adding Gatorade to my diet.

The chemo is very drying and I already had mouth sores the following day of chemo. I continually rinse my mouth with hydrogen peroxide to keep my mouth healthy. The chemo destroys fast growing cells which is why I will be losing my hair. Thus it also damages the mouth and whole intestinal tract. About the fourth day it felt as if my stomach was on fire.

I try to walk on my treadmill twenty minutes at a very slow pace if I feel up to it. That is exhausting as well and I have to monitor my heart rate so it does not get too high. The chemo can also damage the heart as well.

Anyway, I kept focusing on the small picture to get through each minute. Each day grew from minutes to hours to half days which is where I am at physically now. As I said the chemo is very drying, thus my skin now has a new texture and I might add it does do a number on varicose veins as well. I am now searching for patterns forming the state of Indiana on my legs. Needless to say the chemo makes me very nervous/shaky and tired. I consider my day a great success when my shower is done.

I can now say I have one down and three more to go in this first cycle of treatment where I am receiving two chemo drugs before I start my (twelve) one week cycles.

APPENDIX A

My appetite is good after a few days of chemo. I eat several small meals a day to keep the nausea away.

Steve has been wonderful in helping but concern about him taking on the "caretaker" role. I do believe this is somewhat harder on the caretaker at times. Corey is the first to check on me. Clay is still concerned I am going to die. (We have had several talks but he only understands that Grandma had chemo and Grandma still died.)

My head is beginning to itch quite a bit. Can't wait to try my new wig. If and when the hair falls out, it will be 2-3 months after chemo that it should begin to grow again. That would be about November which is when I turn 50. I hope it is not all gray.

I will try to update as I feel up to it. Sometimes it will be days before I get to my computer.

Thanks again for all the positive support, prayers and emails. Marci

PS. As good as I felt yesterday morning, things turned for the worse last night and I had to call my doctor. My blood pressure and heart rate were doing some funky things. Not feeling great this morning but resting is helping.

MARCH FORTH

----- *Original Message* -----
From: *Marci Schmitt*
To: *Undisclosed Recipients*:
Sent: *Thursday, April 16, 2009*
Subject: *Update Apr 15*

Hope everyone had a Happy Easter.

Today is a better day as well as tomorrow will be better than today.

I had my second treatment of the Red Devil Cocktail as they call this particular chemo combo I received on April 7th. Today my head feels a little more attached to my body and I am able to think a little bit. The four days after my chemo treatment are purely "hell" and that is simply put. I simply go into survival mode and try to get by each minute knowing it will be better than the previous one I just went through. It almost seems that the light starts to shine a little on the 4th day. It takes all my energy to get through each minute and force myself to drink the 100 oz of water I need each day to keep the chemo from forming lesions in the kidney and keep myself hydrated. Not to mention to try and eat a bite of something to ward off the nausea. The four days are very nauseating and then it becomes more manageable. It becomes comparable to morning sickness during pregnancy after the 4th day. When it becomes really bad I cry a little and say "AUGUST".

The biggest side effect I have is the way the chemo affects my nervous system. It feels as if my brain is pulling away from my spinal cord and I shake tremendously. My head hurts to think. The 5th, 6th and 7th day my mouth burns to my belly and it seems I fight a mouth sore during this time. Beginning on the 7th day my appetite comes back and I do want to eat something finally. The nausea continues to come and go though.

Some of you have called and left messages after I received chemo. I greatly appreciated the calls and the messages were helpful but I just couldn't even begin to talk. The simple task of talking after chemo is a great struggle and requires a focus that I just don't have at that point. If I am able to answer the phone I will but if I don't it's not that I don't want to talk, I just can't at that point in time. Some of you have left messages of inspiration during this time and believe me they are helpful to hear. Sometimes I replay them from my answering machine.

Anyway, I know each minute will be better than the previous one and the night will be better than this morning and tomorrow will be better than today.

Well when I went to the doctor to receive my second chemo treatment last week, he was quite impressed that I still had my hair. Actually, it was short lived as my hair started coming out in clumps that day. I asked Steve to cut it off so it would not be so messy. (Corey was ok with it but Clay struggled with me losing my hair. He is doing a bit better with it gone now.) I keep a sock hat on my head at home because it is so cold. The wig is very close to my previous hairstyle and I like it so if I have a need to wear it I can. Funny thing about being bald. I have heard so many rumors about how smart a bald person is.

MARCH FORTH

Some of you may already know about this but now that I have experienced this, I can agree (smile)! Of course now we have an increase of bad bald jokes. (If you're bald in front-you're a thinker, if you are bald in back – you're a lover, if you're bald in front and back you're a thoughtful lover and so on.) I think I look like Uncle Walter S. now.

My arm area continues to heal. It is still numb and probably will be for a while. The spring cold fronts, rain fronts are extremely painful to that area. It makes that area feel as if it is drawing up. This also includes the port area as well. . The swelling has gone down enough that I can see the scar area around and under my arm where they took the lymph nodes out. I am still dealing with a tendon under the arm that is causing most of the pain. I continue my stretching so it will lengthen. I am so glad it will be spring and summer as I go through this.

Easter was pleasant for us. It was the first day that I actually had an appetite to eat. (We did not cook as the smells of cooking make me nauseated. My nose is very sensitive to smells.) Steve and the boys went to church and when they got back we ordered from Cracker Barrel because chicken sounded good to me. We distributed the Easter eggs and candy and life was good.

We had some sad news last week concerning Steve's daughter. We pray for her recovery, strength and healing.

Again, Steve has been wonderful with his double duty day. The kids are hanging in there and learning how talented they can be with new chores.

Well next Monday will be my 3rd of my 4th Red Devil Cocktail treatments before I move on to my 15 weekly treatments. I am half way home with that baby.

Again, thank you for all the prayers, emails, phone calls, cards, food etc. It has been extremely helpful to all of us and we greatly appreciate your thoughtfulness, prayers, and concern. As always, I pray for others who are also going through this ordeal.

Marci

----- Original Message -----
From: Marci Schmitt
To: Undisclosed Recipients:
Sent: Thursday, May 14, 2009
Subject: Update May 14th

Hello everyone. I am getting better the further I get away from my last treatment date. A week ago Monday (May 4th) I completed my 4th and final Red Devil Cocktail. Yeah Me! (Just the thought of it makes me nauseated at this point.) This final one was a doosey! I was very much limp and nauseated on the couch for five days. When I finally started coming out of the "hell hole", I realized I had blisters on my lips where my lips met and it felt like a burning torch from my mouth through my whole body to the very bottom. My mouth was so tender that talking formed blisters in my mouth. If I did stand up I was very light headed and at times felt I was going to pass out. I do not want to experience this again and hopefully won't have to in the future and bless those who have to ever go through it. Every side effect lasted longer and twice as strong. It gave the saying "feel the burn" a whole new definition for me.

I made my first attempt Tuesday night to attend a public event (other than doctor appointments and brief stops at the store) in over a month to attend my son's honor's program. I was very exhausted by the end of it and slept soundly for first time since my last good week.

The nausea continues to come and go but is manageable this week. The nausea and the effects on my nervous system make it hard to do some simple tasks. That's why I look so forward to the end of my good (recovery) week so that I can gain some independence again. The better I get sometimes makes me more emotional though as I realize I am getting closer to going in for another treatment. (Chemo makes it hard for your brain to search for words and then say them.)

Driving was not an option in the first week of treatment but is possible towards the end of my good (recovery) week if I plan and rest up to the event.

Next Monday I begin a new treatment with Taxol. I will be treated once a week for 12 weeks. I have been told this is easier to take. Mostly, I hear that it makes your muscles and bones ache but not near the nausea but I'll wait and reserve judgment on it until I have crossed that bridge. I am hoping I will be able to move around a little more and maybe start a little exercise such as walking. We shall see. I miss doing my incline walking on my treadmill and doing my weights.

Hope everyone had a wonderful Mother's Day. I rested the whole day and then Steve, Corey, Clay and I went up to Boonville, picked up my dad and went to the famous Tastee Freeze Ice Cream Shop. The ice cream tasted so wonderful. The coldness soothed my mouth and the creaminess coated my intestinal track. It was actually the first thing that had tasted good all week so I went and got another ice cream cone and life was good. The whole trip lasted a little over an hour. I didn't get out of the car except to sit at the Tastee Freeze and I was so exhausted I came home and rested the evening. It was worth it!

Thanks again for the support and prayers and as always-I keep looking forward.

Love
Marci

----- Original Message -----
From: Marci Schmitt
To: Undisclosed Recipients:
Sent: Friday, June 26, 2009
Subject: Update June 22

Hello everyone. I waited this week to send my update because I am now half way through my Taxol chemo treatment. I have taken six treatments and have six more to go. Next week I will be down to one hand the number of treatments I have left.

This chemo is more doable (if there is a chemo that's doable) in the sense I have little to no nausea. I am able to stand up the next day and talk and do a few things if I pace myself. (As you may recall the last chemo, it took me over a week and a half to accomplish that task.) I am trying to get a small walk in everyday if possible. This chemo still affects my nervous system and makes me shake a lot. My feet and hands feel swollen as if they were stung by several bees. The pads are somewhat numb on my feet and my fingers. I get very bloated after each treatment and my stomach hurts quite a bit on the 3rd-5th day after treatment. The nurse says everyone puts on weight with Taxol. It's the nature of the beast. I am watching this carefully and trying to eat as healthy as I can. But I still seem to gain a little weight every time I go in for my weekly treatment. (I really do not eat junk food; however, I did buy some chocolate chip cookies at Sam's the other day. It's the first time I had a cookie in a long while and chocolate chip are my favorite. It was worth it.) On the 4th and 5th day after treatment, I get somewhat down. I have noticed this pattern and am able to get through this 24-36 hours knowing it will pass. Plus, with the chemo brain I can quickly forget those thoughts that come during that time. I really don't feel well until Sunday comes and then I go in for my treatment on Monday and start the pattern all over again.

This week I am dealing with nosebleeds and nose sores that have developed in my nose. One reason for this is because I have no nose hairs in my nose. (Remember chemo takes out fast growing cells and hair is one of them. These hairs are a buffer to dust pollen etc. and with the chemo my nostril passages are very dry. With that combo you get nose bleeds and nose sores.)

Anyway, I still have the chemo brain where I forget pretty much what I am doing within five seconds of thinking what I thought I was going to do. (Huh?) It makes for a long day. For example, I can walk into the kitchen to get a spoon for my cereal and forget why I walked into the kitchen. Or like people's names while I am talking to them. It can be frustrating but since I forget quickly the frustration doesn't last long. In fact, there is not much I worry about at this point because I forget what I was worrying about. So it does have its advantages. My new motto is the song "Don't Worry, Be Happy! (Cause you can't remember anything anyway.)

Some positives I have had are that I still have about 15% of my hair that Steve shaved off in April. It has grown maybe a quarter of an inch. His comment was it was growing unevenly but I believe it was the cutter who didn't buzz the hair off straight on the initial cut. I still have half of my eyelashes and about half of my eyebrows also. They are thinning but still there. I have kidded my friend about using superglue on them so I can keep my original eyebrows. Anyway, I still have my fingernails. (Some people have lost fingernails during their treatments.) This is why I try to eat so healthy due to the harshness of the chemo. I also realize being in great shape before entering chemo has helped me immensely in the process as well.

Steve continues to support me during my treatments. I know this is tiring for him. He has had to increase his load in running and doing more for the kids and at home as well as continue to work.

He has been great. Corey and Clay continue to help in ways they thought they never could. They have been a big help. We are in the midst of 4H projects and summer camps at this point. I feel more exhaustion since they have been home for summer vacation. It requires a few more steps each day which contributes to my fatigue. My blood counts were below normal this last time and I think this may have contributed towards me making those few extra steps. My numbers have been good throughout treatment so I hope those come up this week. It also would make me feel better as well. It would be nice if we could have a summer vacation. We all need it. Unfortunately, my treatments will be given up to the final week before they go back to school.

Well to wrap it up, other than dealing with the side effects of my nervous system, forgetfulness, nosebleeds, bloating, burning mouth, dry skin and severe exhaustion, I couldn't feel better.

Thanks again for the support and prayers. We truly do appreciate your efforts to help us through this time.

Marci

----- Original Message -----
From: Marci Schmitt
To: Undisclosed Recipients:
Sent: Thursday, July 30, 2009
Subject: update - Jul 30- ONE MORE!

Hello, everyone.

APPENDIX A

Just wanted to drop a quick line to update everyone. The fog is starting to clear (not in my brain yet) and the end is in sight. I now have ONE more treatment left and I will be finished with my chemo sessions. What began in March will end this August 3rd-my last and 16th chemo treatment. As I get closer to this date especially this week, the exhaustion of persevering through each treatment is coming to a conclusion. I have been so fixated on the present moment to not look behind or ahead but just survive the moment. I will be looking forward to moving from a mental state of survival to healing and recovery.

Some things I am looking forward to:

<u>My hair.</u> It is starting to grow on my head even though I am still 90% bald. In some places it is a half inch. I ask certain individuals if it is blonde or gray. They tell me it is blonde. I don't know if they are being kind or blind.

<u>Nose hair.</u> Just so that it will help keep moisture in my nose and the nosebleeds will stop. (Just stopping the chemo so I can keep moisture in my body would be such a thrill.)

<u>Eyelashes and eyebrows.</u> I just have a few. They suddenly all fell out over night about three weeks ago. (I forgot to add the superglue.)

<u>Fingernails.</u> About half of my fingernails are dying and pulling away at the ends of my fingers. It hurts to grasp things.

Feeling in my feet. The bottoms of my feet feel as if they are half asleep.

Muscles that don't ache. My legs and arms hurt to move. They burn and ache with every movement I make. It has been non-stop for the last two weeks. (A new reference to "feel the burn").

No blisters in my throat mouth and stomach. Just plain and simple - this hurts all the time. (This is the old but new reference to "feel the burn".)

No more nausea. No explanation there.

No more headaches and lightheadedness.

No more dry skin - I look and feel (I think) like an elephant.

Losing the 10-15 lbs I put on. I hope most will be gone due to the chemo. My stomach is so bloated it feels like I am about six months pregnant. This will help when I stop taking the steroids.

My strength. I know getting older makes us tired but this exhaustion is a little too much.

My nervous system to calm down. Having my balance return and hands stop shaking will be a blessing.

My short term memory. Wow can't wait for that. It was rough when I would forget the person's name I was talking to or like *the time I left the gas grill on because I forgot to turn it off when I was done.*

<u>But most of all a clean bill of health.</u> After I receive my last chemo treatment, I will start a series of tests all over to make sure the cancer did not grow in other places or was resistant to the chemo. I hope this will be an end to the side effects and beginning of the healing process. I am still fortunate that I still only have a FEW side effects. Some people have harsher ones such as the chemo giving them leukemia.

Again, we want to thank everyone for their support through this journey. I have had many people tell me this has been an educational experience and had no idea what people went through during their chemo. Writing emails has been therapy for me and helped me stay focused on dealing and going forward with this bump. I can't thank you enough for those who have emailed, sent cards or called at the time I needed it most. Steve, Corey, Clay and I thank each of you for your support and prayers that you have given us. Thank you.

And so it goes, if you still ask me how I feel or how I am doing- I will still tell you - terrific!

God Bless,
Marci

----- *Original Message* -----
From: <u>*Marci Schmitt*</u>
To: <u>*Undisclosed Recipients:*</u>
Sent: Monday, August 3, 2009
Subject: update Aug 3rd

Hello, everyone. I have great news. I went to the doctor today to receive my last chemo treatment. After my visit, the doctor cancelled my last treatment because my side effects I am experiencing throughout my body were too severe to warrant any positive gain with any more treatment. Good news is I have no more treatments. (Bad news is my nervous system, muscles and feet are not in good shape among other things in my body.) I now have a whole week that I am ahead in my healing schedule. In three weeks I begin another series of tests to determine if we did any good with the chemo. I am expecting good results. I still have a ways to go to feel physically well but mentally I am slowly feeling relief.

Marci

----- *Original Message* -----
From: <u>*Marci Schmitt*</u>
Sent: Wednesday, August 26, 2009
Subject: Re: Fingers crossed

I am so exhausted it is unbelievable. I took my Dad to the doctor today. . . . It was the first time I have taken him since February. It exhausted me. I came home and took a nap and slept three hours. Guess I need it. I'm like a little puppy going and then suddenly I fall over and go to sleep.

I'm not sure when I will feel like visitors. Every day I get stronger than the last. My house is a mess. (Not that that would keep me from inviting you.) I have a lot of cleaning and sorting to do. I just have to laugh about it but it seems that they (my family) have put a bowl in every cabinet I have. I can't find a lot of things in the kitchen because they would put things "away" if you know what I mean. I finally went up to the boys' rooms and couldn't find the floor in either room. I have not been able to go up and check if you know what I mean. I just walked back downstairs. . . . I have had a hard time sleeping on my bed. The chemo has every muscle in my body hurting and burning so I end up sleeping on the soft couch. . . . I want to hurry up and be healthy. But when I look back I know I have made giant strides. I've been told six months to a year before I feel like myself again. It would be nice to see you before then but I just don't know when to tell you.

Take care and enjoy your time with your sons before they go (to school).

Marci

----- Original Message -----
From: Marci Schmitt
To: Undisclosed Recipients:
Sent: Tuesday, August 25, 2009
Subject: Good News so far

MARCH FORTH

Hello Everyone,

I have good news to report. Yesterday I went to see the doctor about the results of my CT scan. As far as they can determine, my scan is clear. (Notice that they never say cancer free.) Anyway, this is good news for the Schmitt Family. The next plan of action is to do follow up testing and monitoring for the next few months. I am almost giddy to know I do not have to go through chemo at this point. I will be taking some preventive pills for the next five years and of course do the x-ray, scans etc. peppered in along the way. Presently, I am going through physical therapy to help my arm and shoulder around my mastectomy site. This is helping me tremendously.

Each day I feel a little better than I did the day before. I still have some lingering side effects that I am still dealing with (exhaustion, numb feet, muscle aches, stomach to mouth problems) but my hair and eyelashes are starting to grow. My fingernails are growing again. My nose bleeds have finally stopped. My skin is FINALLY producing oil again. (Such little things we take for granted.) I am able to do a little more each day. Friday, I will be getting my chemo port removed. That will be a major celebration in itself to be free of that item that has been lodged in my chest. My chemo brain is doing better. (What a number the chemo has done to my short term memory.)

As with anyone who has been thru this ordeal, I feel I am sitting on the other side of the fence looking at the same world but feeling a little different. Even though I am on that side of the fence, I am so thankful I can still see that world especially with my family.

Again, thanks for all your support and prayers. We very much appreciate it. Thanks for letting me sound off through these emails. It was very much my therapy.

Thanks, again.
Marci

As I have said many times, writing and e-mailing my thoughts and updates was my therapy. Many people were reaching out to me when they responded back to these updates. Each time someone would e-mail me, pray for me, or call, it lifted me and helped me to focus on the finish. Never under-estimate the slightest good intention when dealing with someone who has been diagnosed with cancer and is succumbing to the rigorous chemotherapy sessions and doctor visits. It all helps and your thoughtfulness is greatly magnified for the person who is on the receiving end.

I have to share some of my favorite e-mail replies to my updates. Although some individuals did not respond, they helped in other ways to make sure I knew they were there for me during my journey. Some would just respond "hang in there." I wish I could print them all but for now have selected certain e-mails that would help anyone who is presently going through cancer treatments. Simply put, I surrounded myself with positive people and cannot say enough about all of them.

MARCH FORTH

Congratulations!

Marci,
You have been so strong through this ordeal and I know as well as you, it's been the Lord carrying you and holding your hand every step of the way, saying don't give up my child. I just don't know if I would handle this situation as well as you have, if I were in your shoes.

I found out about a lady who used to attend our church, had a double mastectomy last Friday. I believe she only had the cancer in one breast, but with doctor recommendations, she decided to have both removed. I don't know if you know her, but she's in her early 40's, always appeared to be healthy and active, a Christ follower. It makes me wonder why. I feel the same way about you. I don't feel God gave you or her this disease, but I do believe God is always there to get you through it if you call on Him. PTL for that!

I'm looking forward to reporting the good news to my small group tonight. We love to hear the praises from the good works of our God!

Thank you, Jesus for watching over Marci and her family.

We give you all the glory and the praise! Continue to give her physical strength, mental alertness, and ease every pain in her body. Thank you for the great reports from the tests. I ask that you will put a hedge around Marci to keep her cancer free. Lord, send a special blessing down to Steve and her sons. We understand that they go through so much as well during this time and how strong they need to be, to be there for Marci to take care of her physical needs and lift her up when it seems like there is no end in sight. Jesus, help me and others know that we should never take even the smallest of things for granted. Make us wise in knowing what we really should be thankful for. Lord God, be with ------ and her family. We know your mighty works. Thank you again for all you do and all you've done!

In Jesus' Name we pray, AMEN!

I'll close for now. I'm always thinking about you and looking forward to seeing you soon around the pop ice or the popcorn machine.

Your friend,
N-----

----- Original Message -----
From: <u>Marci Schmitt</u>
Sent: Saturday, August 29, 2009
Subject: Re: Good News so far

Thanks -----. We already had a bump this week. The doctor

wanted to do more surgery but after further review we will stay in a holding pattern and hope for the best.

Marci

----- Original Message -----
From: ------
Sent: Monday, September 14, 2009
Subject: Team Marci - Race for the Cure - This Saturday, September 19, 2009!

Staff:
Thanks to all employees, family members, and friends who joined our team in the "Race for the Cure." We have named our team in honor of Marci Schmitt, Steve Schmitt's wife. During 2009 Marci was diagnosed with breast cancer. She underwent surgery and then several rounds of chemotherapy. We are happy to update you that Marci is now on her road to recovery.

Every year millions of women are diagnosed with this deadly disease. We realize due to family obligations, work obligations, or health reasons, not all employees could join us in our walk for the cure. However, we are asking you at this time to consider a monetary donation to help fight for a cure and support one of our own. You can go to the home page for "Race for the Cure", www.Komenevansville.org, and make an on-line donation to our team, "Team Marci" or I can submit a check or cash in your behalf. Whatever you feel comfortable donating would be greatly appreciated or if that is not an option at this time, we are asking you to support Steve, Marci and family with your thoughts and prayers. Please forward this information to all your team members.

Thank you.

--- Original Message -----
From: Marci Schmitt
Sent: Wednesday, September 02, 2009
Subject: Re: how are you?

Yesterday I started coming down with a cold of all things. Feel fortunate that I never once got sick during the chemo.

Well to make a long story short, I got a clear test last Monday. Then the doctor called on Wednesday wanting to go back and do more surgery and take more lymph nodes based on a study that came out in June. If you remember I had one positive node found not during surgery but on the pathology report. At that time no more lymph nodes were going to be removed because the tumor was still encapsulated. After talking with ------ , my doctor and I came to the agreement since the tumor was still encapsulated, it would probably do more harm to me to remove more lymph nodes because of the lymphedema problems, etc.

As you can see it was a no win situation. Remove lymph nodes, more problems. If the lymph nodes were negative I would be strapped with problems on my arm. If they were positive why the hell did I go through chemo for six months? Since the node was encapsulated this was the selling point to sit tight and test in three months etc. and hope the chemo killed all the cancer cells. I have to stay in menopause and will be tested monthly. I went into menopause because of the chemo. If I come out of menopause I have to take my ovaries out. I am now on ------ to help my body not make estrogen. I should be on this for about five years. Doing physical therapy on my arm and that is helping with some pain.

...See ya later and thanks for asking. It really does help me. Marci

----- Original Message -----
From: Marci Schmitt
Sent: Thursday, September 17, 2009
Subject: Re: Team Marci for the Komen Race for the Cure

So sorry to hear of the deaths in your family. Hope you are recovering/adjusting and please know I am thinking of you and your family.

I feel lucky first and foremost. I am extremely tired but that is getting better but not fast enough. My fingernails are 3/4 dead but new ones are coming on at the bottoms. My eyelashes are really starting to grow as well as my eyebrows. (They all fell off a couple of weeks ago. I woke up and they were gone.) My feet are a little numb but doable. My throat and stomach still bother me. They are irritated because I just did not have any mucus to coat them. My hair is coming in. I still have a little bald spot on top (think too much) but it is about 1/4-1/2 inch in spots. My skin is covered in bumps which are my glands starting to produce oil again. The biggest problem I have at this point is my muscles. I feel like a Mack truck has run me over. Every little muscle down to my fingers aches. I am told this takes 6-12 months to get over. That is one reason I was taking steroids with my chemo to help with that but now I am not taking anything and it is a lingering effect. I try to exercise to overcome pain and tiredness. I'm doing pretty well with that- not sure sometimes to push or rest. My bed feels so hard so I double over one of those temporpedic memory foam mattresses on my bed. It helps a little. I usually get up at night a couple of hours and then go to bed again. I feel lucky I did not have to do more. Some random thoughts (like I'm gonna die!) do enter my mind but I try to quickly extinguish those. I am here today and that is what counts.

As far as lunch, I am not quite there yet. I am trying to add more activity daily and will do well with that then I will regress for a couple of days. I am so tired! If I feel like lunch maybe I can call you at the last minute or something. Otherwise it probably will be October before I can get there. I am running quite a bit with the kids' activities and take rests twice a day so I can gear up for that in the evening. Slowly but surely, I am getting there. I am looking forward to lunch with you. I haven't talked to you in a while.

Marci

MARCH FORTH

----- *Original Message* -----
From: <u>Marci Schmitt</u>
Sent: Wednesday, September 30, 2009
Subject: Re: give me an update

Hi -----. Thanks for asking. I am doing so much better. The only lingering effects I have right now are I tire easily but my rest is so sound now. My fingernails are half dead but showing growth midway in the fingernail. My mouth and throat are still not healed and will be doing an endoscopy in two weeks. It looks like I still have lesions down in my throat. My hair, eyebrows, and eyelashes are starting to grow very fast as well as my oil glands are starting to gel. This will help my dry skin. I try to exercise when I can and I am becoming stronger every day. I am still focused on recovery and tend to break down crying a little more because I sometimes think about what I just went through. But that's part of my healing mentally.

Chemo put me in menopause and that is where they are trying to keep me. I am taking a pill to prevent me from making estrogen (because estrogen was feeding my cancer). I have hot flashes several times a day. If I come out of menopause they will have to remove my ovaries. Only 10% return to premenopausal state after chemo so my odds are good I won't. We play odds all day with our life don't we?

Both boys are playing football so we have been busy shuffling to and from practices and games. Take care. Hope all is well.

Marci

APPENDIX A

From: <u>Marci Schmitt</u>
Sent: Friday, October 23, 2009
Subject: Re:

I am doing much better but very, very tired. It's all I can do to keep up with my kids and my Dad. I will go for my three month check up on November 16th. Thanks for asking. I really do appreciate it.

Marci

----- Original Message -----
From: <u>Marci Schmitt</u>
To: <u>Undisclosed Recipients</u>:
Sent: Tuesday, November 17, 2009
Subject: Great news

I went to the doctor today and received great news. My three month pet/ct scan was clear and I am good to go for another six months. My bone density scan was a little low (probably from the chemo) but I can hopefully fix that with some calcium supplements. Now I feel like I really have something to celebrate for my 50th birthday at the end of this month. Woo Hoo!! Bet you never heard of someone looking so forward to that!!!!

Thanks for the encouraging words and prayers.

God Bless.
Marci

MARCH FORTH

----- *Original Message* -----
From: Marci Schmitt
Sent: Friday, December 11, 2009
Subject: Re: . . . update

I have been thinking of you all week. I knew you were coming up on your surgery. I have been extremely busy celebrating my "50" birthday, my good news, getting ready for Christmas and attending my two boys' basketball games. I am trying to get to my "fast" pace I used to be at but am not keeping up as I am tired. I am so slow at getting things done. Was looking at the mug you gave me this week. Anyway, I hope to call you maybe this weekend.

So good to hear that your scan and density tests were OK. As you may recall, my bone scan was negative and I have osteopenia. Trying to increase my calcium as much as possible. Have been having trouble with the ------ too. My joints, especially my larger ones - shoulders, hips and knees-have been killing me. My muscles ache extremely all the way down to my fingers. I also have some spots of my bones that ache as well. Had to call the doctor and ask because it was so painful I could hardly move. Felt like my last few weeks of chemo in every way. "Complained" at last appointment about joints hurting. . . . Anyway the nurse talked with (the doctor) and said I could try ------. I told her I was a pretty tough cookie to tough it out if needed but just wanted to know if I had to put up with this type of pain for five years or if I had some reaction that was more than it should be. She said sometimes it gets better. Told her I would finish prescription and see. ------ could be worse.

At least I am not nauseated. Anyway, got on the internet and found these systems were extremely common. (You know I gotta read!) Today is a better day.

Had my mammogram this week. They looked at spots that were bothering me this summer. The nurse tends to think it was maybe a tendon or ligament. They all felt it was OK so I got through that hurdle. Besides, my mammograms are half price now! (smile)

. . . have good holidays. Take Care.
Marci

----- Original Message -----
From: Marci Schmitt
To: bethelucc.org
Sent: Monday, December 21, 2009
Subject: Thank you for Bethel January Record

Can you please put the following thank you in the January Bethel Record? -Thanks.

We would like to thank our Bethel Church friends and members for their support during my illness this past year. We would like to thank you for the cards, food and most importantly the prayers we received during my surgery and chemo treatments. We felt truly blessed and thankful for your support. Even though each day still presents some lingering challenges from the chemo treatments and the medicine I am presently taking, I continue to gain my strength back daily. This event has truly been a walk with God. Recently, I received results that my initial scans are clear of cancer. This is good news! We continue to hope and pray for good results in 2010 and beyond.

Thanks, again.
Marci Schmitt Family

I cannot thank enough my friends and members of Bethel UCC Church who prayed for us and brought food for our family.

----- *Original Message* -----
From: Marci Schmitt
Sent: Thursday, January 21, 2010
Subject: Re: Cancer

I am sure you are in shock as I was and still am. I'm sure you have lots of questions about life sitting in front of you just as I did. Just remember now is all we got and take it one day at a time. I will put you on my prayer list. Keep me informed, OK? They can do so much and it sounds like you are on top of it. I have a friend who had that and she is still going great.

I am doing better. I am extremely tired all the time. It is just indescribable. I drop down like a worn out puppy. My joints and muscles ache a lot. Sometimes I feel I can't get out of bed. I want to cry and do at times. Part of it is the healing process and the other part is side effects of my medicine. The good part is I have to keep moving so it won't hurt as bad but it hurts to move. Anyway, everyone says my color looks good but I feel about 60%. My hair is about 1½" long now. I love combing it. It is such the small things in life.

However, I do want to correct one thing. I do not have cancer anymore. The mastectomy and chemo killed it! Healing can be a mental thing. Like the book said, you can't have a negative thought. Tell yourself things are not going to get worse!!!!!!!!!!!! OK?

Take care,
Marci

----- Original Message -----
From: Marci Schmitt
To: Undisclosed Recipients:
Sent: Wednesday, May 19, 2010
Subject: Update

Many of you have been asking lately how I have been. I am getting stronger, growing lots of curly hair; continue to have joint and muscle pain and tiredness. Each day is slowly but surely getting better. I have come a long way since March and especially since last August.

This past Monday I went in for my six months pet/ct scan. Today I went in for my three month doctor visit and to get results of my pet/ct scan. After sitting in the lobby crying all morning, I have good news. The scan is clear. I will have another follow up visit in August.

Thanks again for all your prayers and support.
Marci

----- Original Message -----
From: <u>Marci Schmitt</u>
Sent: Sunday, May 30, 2010
Subject: Re:

Glad to hear from you. I was a basket case this time waiting for my scan. When I came back two days later (after my scan) to the doctor's office for the results, I walked into the doctor's office door and started crying. . . . I tried to stop crying but I couldn't. Finally, I went to the restroom to try and collect myself and came back and sat down and cried again. I just could not stop crying. Steve was focused on my appointment time. He was wondering if the nurses forgot me. They were taking patients that had arrived after my sign in. . . . I said maybe it's because my scan was bad and they were leaving me for last before lunch. . . . Finally, they called my name and I went back there and just bawled the whole time I was getting my vitals. I finally just quit holding it in. I cried down the hall to the doctor office. I cried when the doctor came in. I cried. Of course my scan was OK. He asked me how I had been and I just said I have been so emotional the last two months. It has been awful. The doctor asked me if he thought it was me facing what has happened the last year and I said I think so. Finally, I am crying now. I am so emotional and I hate it. I had a lady come up to me after my doctor's visit and she told me she hated seeing me crying in the lobby and hoped everything was OK and wished me the best. Yikes! I was trying not to be noticeable. Oh well. I thanked her and told her all was well. I was talking to ----- the other night and told her I feel like I am detached. I am so sick of the pain blah blah blah.

But.......................! I am here and I am getting better every day. We have come so far especially you. I don't know how you do it—working, etc. I try to keep walking and doing my weights. I think I am finally starting to get some things done that I have been trying to do for the past six years (when I quit work).

Things are progressing and then they go backwards for me mentally now. I am swinging all over the place on my emotions and I know that but I still can't control them. . . . People who have not physically gone through this have no clue. . . .

Well this email sounds so down doesn't it? Sorry about that but I guess I am venting. Anyway, did you read the article about the aromatase inhibitors? They are using them to reduce tumors before any type of surgery. (Gotta read you know.) They are reducing tumors so much that mastectomies are being eliminated. They either eliminate the tumor or reduce the surgery to lumpectomies. It also is reducing the use of chemo. They are having great success with it. We should feel comforted that we are taking that "pill" and knowing it really is helping us. I am still aching from joint and muscle pain and dryness all over though. Who would have thought it would take this long to heal?

. . . Hope you had a great weekend on the lake. You deserve it. Please take care of yourself. You are doing great! I have

confidence that things are going well for you. Keep those nega-
tive thoughts away from your mind. I am sorry for your friend
and I know that weighs in the back of your mind for you as
well. It does me too but we cannot let those negative thoughts
come into our mind. We and everybody else only have today.

Anyway, I will stop this marathon email and hope to see you
soon.

Take care,
Marci

----- Original Message -----
From: Marci Schmitt
To: Undisclosed Recipients:
Sent: Saturday, October 02, 2010 8:19 PM
Subject: good news bad news

The good news was the spot they were looking at was a benign
fibroadenoma. But the bad news was they found the Atypical
Lobular Hyperplasia Cells behind the fibroadenoma. I had the
MRI because I was having pain in the breast. The MRI re-
sults did not show anything where I felt the pain but did find
this other mass (the fibroadenoma). When they biopsied the fi-
broadenoma, it was OK but then they found the atypical cells
while finding the fibroadenoma. In a long roundabout way they
found the atypical cells.

Anyway, Atypical Lobular Hyperplasia cells are not consid-
ered cancer at this point. Basically, the cells are abnormal and

sometimes it takes 10-15 years to turn into cancer. Sometimes they do not turn into cancer. Sometimes they treat it with medication. Sometimes they take the cells out to find a tumor attached. Anyway, I have to have the cells removed. This is why I need to see a surgeon which is scheduled on the 19th. Since they found these cells, considering my history, and since I have to have lumpectomy surgery, I am considering a mastectomy on the right side. I will know more after the visit with the surgeon on October 19th.

After all I have been through and when you're in this position, a person is always waiting for the hammer to fall again. Well it fell but did not knock me out this time. We are well ahead of the game and things are going pretty good. I am still getting stronger each month. I do appreciate the prayers and hope soon we can find an answer for this dreaded disease.

Hope everyone is still having a good weekend.
Marci A. Schmitt

----- Original Message -----
From: Marci Schmitt
To: Undisclosed Recipients:
Sent: Wednesday, October 20, 2010
Subject: Surgeon visit and follow-up

I know many of you are waiting to hear my results from the surgeon visit yesterday. I still do not have a definitive answer where we are going with this and waiting to get all the information needed to make a decision. I am waiting on an oncologist to get back with me to discuss further.

Again, this is NOT CLASSIFIED AS CANCER OR PRECANCEROUS! However, it warrants my attention due to my past history and age of previous diagnosis. (See, I am still considered young for some things in life! :)

If anyone else had this diagnosis they may very well ignore it. One day it may be there and one day it may not. It is hard to explain in an email. That's why I am waiting for all my info to make the best decision that is right for me and my case. There is no rush for action or decision. I have plenty of time to decide unlike last time.

I will return to the surgeon in two weeks for a follow-up. I appreciate everyone's thoughts and prayers and will let everyone know something when I have all the medical advice given to me.

Thanks again for the prayers and support. (Hope I have everyone on this email as I had to redo my group.)

Marci A. Schmitt

-----Original Message-----
From: Marci Schmitt
To: Undisclosed Recipients:
Sent: Tue, Oct 26, 2010
Subject: Surgery November 1st

All,

After discussing my options with my surgeon and oncologist, I will be having the second mastectomy. Surgery is scheduled this Monday, November 1st.

*This surgery will be labeled as **the drive by whack a boob surgery** II!*

*Are you all sitting? Good. This surgery will be **done as out-patient surgery** in an ambulatory facility next to the hospital. (What is this world coming to?!)*

*Again, thank you all for your concern, prayers and support. I am trying to digest not the surgery but that it will be done as **outpatient** surgery.*

Marci

-----Original Message-----
From: <u>Marci Schmitt</u>
To: <u>Undisclosed Recipients</u>:
Sent: Wed, November 10, 2010
Subject: update

Just to update you all. Surgery was completed on November 1st. This was a definite drive by surgery. Actually had to walk to surgery room and lay down on the surgery table. Afterwards given pain medicine and moved to a recliner. Pain meds were given upon waking, then morphine shortly after that. Had a reaction to the morphine. Still in pain— gave me Percocet. This made my heart race so they gave me a Valium. By the time I got home (three hours later and after the hour and a half surgery), I took half a Phenergan because my stomach was upset, followed by two Lortab. 48 hours later, I took myself off the pain medicine. (Wasn't in that much pain.) I called the doctor because I was still nauseous and anxious. My lungs and nervous system were burning and shaking. I truly believe I had a reaction to the anesthesia. Anyway, they told me I was suffering anxiety and to get some Xanax! Whatever! Got the Xanax on Friday and took a half of a pill at night. I slept good but lungs still burning and nervous system still shaking. This is still bothering me but slowly but surely going away. I knew it was not anxiety. (Anxiety doesn't make you nauseous or your lungs burn. Although that half of the pill does give me a good night's sleep!)

Yesterday went to the doctor to get the drain tube out. Pathology report was good. No more treatment necessary at this time. Will get the 24 metal staples out on Friday. Mental pain more than physical pain at this time and like all things will get better with time.

Next week is my six month checkup with oncologist.

For now I feel great in the first hour after waking from a restful night. Then I get very light headed and weak and need to lie down. I don't have the energy to walk because I feel so light headed.

Thank you all for your support and prayers.
Marci A. Schmitt

APPENDIX A

-----*Original Message*-----
From: <u>*Marci Schmitt*</u>
To: <u>*Undisclosed Recipients*</u>:
Date: Sun, 21 Nov 2010

Just to let you all know, I am still recuperating and getting stronger post surgery. Again my path report was clear on mastectomy on November 1st. Went for six month checkup for initial diagnosis this past week and it was also clear. Good to go for 2011. Again, thank you for all of your support and prayers for me and my family. I am a lucky one. Please pray and support those who may not be.

Please have a wonderful Thanksgiving. Please pray for our troops who allow us to celebrate this and the rest of the Christmas and Holiday season.
Thanks.
Marci

APPENDIX B
FOOTNOTES

1. Pam Stephan, "Types of Breast Reconstruction,"BreastCancer.About.com Guide, updated April 15, 2010.
2. American Cancer Society, www.cancer.org; National Cancer Institute, www.cancer.gov; Harris, J.R., Lippman, M.E., Morrow, M., Osborne, C.K., eds. *Diseases of the Breast.* Lippincott, Williams & Wilkins, 4th ed. 2010.
3. Ibid.
4. Ibid.
5. Breastcancer.org/Symptoms & Diagnosis/Types of Breast Cancer/Male Breast Cancer, July 18, 2009.
6. American Cancer Society; National Cancer Institute; Lippman et al.
7. Ibid.
8. Ibid.
9. Pam Stephan, "Invasive Lobular Carcinoma—ILC Breast Cancer," BreastCancer.About.com,

updated July 24, 2008.

10. Ibid.

11. Maureen Salamon, "How Breast Cancer Spreads (Early Detection and Improved Treatments Help Increase Survival Rates)," BreastCancer.About. com, July, 2008.

12. Ibid.

The information above was accurate at the time this book went to press.

CPSIA information can be obtained at www.ICGtesting.com
Printed in the USA
BVOW081635171012

303220BV00002BA/25/P